KT-496-354

CLINICAL FINALS AND HOW TO PASS THEM

OSCEs, short cases and long cases

Commissioning Editor: Laurence Hunter
Project Development Manager: Janice Urquhart
Project Manager: Frances Affleck
Designer: Erik Bigland

CLINICAL FINALS
AND HOW TO PASS THEM
OSCEs, short cases and long cases

KEVIN P HANRETTY MD FRCOG
Consultant Obstetrician and
 Gynaecologist
The Queen Mother's Hospital
Glasgow UK

TOM TURNER FRCP
Consultant Paediatrician
The Royal Hospital for Sick
 Children
Glasgow UK

JOHN R McGREGOR MD FRCS
Consultant Surgeon
Crosshouse Hospital
Kilmarnock UK

STUART HOOD MD MRCP
Consultant Cardiologist
Royal Alexandra Hospital
Paisley UK

ROBERT HUNTER MD FRCPsych
Consultant Psychiatrist
Gartnavel Royal Hospital
Glasgow UK

SECOND EDITION

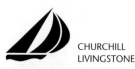

CHURCHILL
LIVINGSTONE

EDINBURGH   LONDON   NEW YORK   OXFORD   PHILADELPHIA
ST LOUIS   SYDNEY   TORONTO   2004

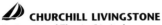

CHURCHILL LIVINGSTONE

An imprint of Elsevier Limited

© 2004, Elsevier Limited. All rights reserved.

The right of Kevin P. Hanretty, Tom Turner, John R. McGregor, Stuart Hood and Robert Hunter to be identified as authors of this work has been asserted by them in accordance with the Copyright, Designs and Patents Act 1988

No part of this publication may be reproduced, stored in a retrieval system, or transmitted in any form or by any means, electronic, mechanical, photocopying, recording or otherwise, without either the prior permission of the publishers or a licence permitting restricted copying in the United Kingdom issued by the Copyright Licensing Agency, 90 Tottenham Court Road, London W1T 4LP. Permissions may be sought directly from Elsevier's Health Sciences Rights Department in Philadelphia, USA: phone: (+1) 215 238 7869, fax: (+1) 215 238 2239, e-mail: healthpermissions@elsevier.com. You may also complete your request on-line via the Elsevier Science homepage (http://www.elsevier.com), by selecting 'Customer Support' and then 'Obtaining Permissions'.

First edition 1998
Second edition 2004

ISBN 0 443 07359 7

British Library Cataloguing in Publication Data
A catalogue record for this book is available from the British Library

Library of Congress Cataloging in Publication Data
A catalog record for this book is available from the Library of Congress

Notice
Medical knowledge is constantly changing. Standard safety precautions must be followed, but as new research and clinical experience broaden our knowledge, changes in treatment and drug therapy may become necessary or appropriate. Readers are advised to check the most current product information provided by the manufacturer of each drug to be administered to verify the recommended dose, the method and duration of administration, and contraindications. It is the responsibility of the practitioner, relying on experience and knowledge of the patient, to determine dosages and the best treatment for each individual patient. Neither the Publisher nor the authors assume any liability for any injury and/or damage to persons or property arising from this publication.
The Publisher

ELSEVIER

your source for books, journals and multimedia in the health sciences

www.elsevierhealth.com

LYMINGTON HOSPITAL LIBRARY

The Publisher's policy is to use **paper manufactured from sustainable forests**

Printed in China

PREFACE

This is the second edition of *Clinical Finals*. The first edition resulted from a perceived reduction in the opportunities for students to develop the specific techniques required to pass clinical examinations. In particular, the authors saw the need for a handbook which would aid students in their preparation for the problem-based approach required for clinical examinations.

This new edition has resulted from a further development in undergraduate education, namely, the widespread introduction of objective structured clinical examinations or OSCEs. The text has been thoroughly revised to take into account the techniques required in order to be successful in this type of examination. The other substantial change has been the introduction of a section on psychiatry. Psychiatry now forms a part of finals examinations in many medical schools and this addition is timely.

Finally, as before, it is hoped that this handbook may help students to develop their talents in order to achieve the principal aim of being good doctors.

Glasgow 2004   K. P. H.

CONTENTS

4. GYNAECOLOGY 189

7. PSYCHIATRY

COMMONLY USED ABBREVIATIONS

ABG	arterial blood gas
ABPI	Ankle brachial pressure index
ACE	angiotensin-converting enzyme
AD	Alzheimer's disease
ADL	activities of daily living
AF	atrial fibrillation
ALT	alanine aminotransferase
AMI	acute myocardial infarction
APH	antepartum haemorrhage
APTT	acrivated partial thromboplastin time
AST	aspartate aminotransferase
AV	arteriovenous
AVM	arteriovenous malformation
BD	twice a day (Latin *bis die*)
BMI	body mass index
BP	blood pressure
CAPD	continuous ambulatory peritoneal dialysis
CBT	cognitive behaviour therapy
CCF	congestive cardiac failure
CIN	cervical intraepithelial neoplasia
CJD	Creutzfeldt–Jakob disease
CMP	case management plan
CNS	central nervous system
COPD	chronic obstructive pulmonary disease
CRP	C-reactive protein
CSF	cerebrospinal fluid
CT	computed tomography

COMMONLY USED ABBREVIATIONS

CT	connective tissue
CVA	cerebrovascular accident
CVP	central venous pressure
CVS	cardiovascular system
CXR	chest X-ray
DIP	distal interphalangeal (joint)
DM	diabetes mellitus
DMARD	disease-modifying anti-rheumatic drugs
DS	disseminated sclerosis
DVT	deep vein thrombosis
ECG	electrocardiogram
EEG	electroencephalogram
EPO	erythropoietin
ERCP	endoscopic retrograde cholangiopancreatography
ESR	erythrocyte sedimentation rate
FBC	full blood count
FNAC	fine needle aspiration cytology
FOB	faecal occult blood
GGT	gamma glutamyl transferase
GI	gastrointestinal
GTT	glucose tolerance test
HIV	human immunodeficiency virus
HPV	human papilloma virus
HRT	hormone replacement therapy
HSV	herpes simplex virus
IBD	inflammatory bowel disease
IHD	ischaemic heart disease
IUGR	intrauterine growth restriction
IV	intravenous

JVP	jugular venous pressure
LBBB	left bundle branch block
LBD	Lewy body dementia
LFTs	liver function tests
LMN	lower motor neurone
LV	left ventricle
LVF	left ventricular failure
LVH	left ventricular hypertrophy
MCV	mean corpuscular volume
MI	myocardial infarction
MMSE	Mini Mental State Examination
MND	motor neurone disease
MRI	magnetic resonance imaging
MS	multiple sclerosis
MSE	mental state examination
NSAID	non-steroidal anti-inflammatory drug
OA	osteoarthritis
OCD	obsessive–compulsive disorder
OSCE	objective structured clinical examination
PA	pernicious anaemia
PD	Parkinson's disease
PIP	proximal interphalangeal (joint)
PMB	postmenopausal bleeding
PMH	past medical history
PPH	postpartum haemorrhage
PPROM	preterm premature rupture of the membranes
PR	per rectum
PT	prothrombin time
PV	per vaginam
QID	four times a day (Latin *quater in die*)

RA	rheumatoid arthritis
RV	right ventricle
RVH	right ventricular hypertrophy
SAH	subarachnoid haemorrhage
SFD	small for dates
SLE	systemic lupus erythematosus
TB	tuberculosis
TFTs	thyroid function tests
TIA	transient ischaemic attack
TPN	total parenteral nutrition
TSH	thyroid-stimulating hormone
UC	ulcerative colitis
UMN	upper motor neurone
UTI	urinary tract infection
U&Es	urea and electrolytes
VE	vaginal examination
WCC	white cell count

INTRODUCTION

Clinical and oral examinations form a fundamental part of the assessment of your competence at every stage of your clinical training. Unfortunately, the performance of candidates in clinical final examinations can sometimes be poor and, ironically, the performance in clinicals and orals often does not reflect either knowledge or competence.

You will already have encountered colleagues who do well in written examinations but badly when presented with a real patient. Alternatively, you meet people who come out of an examination and complain about how difficult either the cases or the examiners were, when neither is necessarily true. In undergraduate examinations the examiners' aim is to identify that you have met the standards required to practise as a doctor in the supervised post of junior house officer. This is a taxing responsibility for the examiners. However, it is important to remember that they are really trying to pass you rather than fail you. You will become bored by the number of times people tell you this, but it is actually true. In other words, defeat in the final MB examination usually results from 'own goals' rather than enormously difficult cases.

All students should be able to pass their clinical exams. Acceptance into medical school should mean that you certainly have the intellectual capacity. Why is it, therefore, that some candidates still fail? One answer is simply lack of effort, but we will assume you are not in that category. Basically, success depends

1

on learning the techniques of presentation peculiar to clinical exams. The purpose of this handbook is to help with how you might do this. It is not a textbook and not intended as such, but consists of a general introduction to the aspects of history and examination particular to each of the principal disciplines in the finals: medicine, surgery, obstetrics and gynaecology, paediatrics and psychiatry. For each specialty there then follows a number of cases with which you might be presented in the finals.

One current problem for students is that different medical schools, and even specialties within schools, may use different methods to assess students. Within specialties the examination may be on a single long case, a series of short cases or structured orals. The last may be part of an OSCE (objective structured clinical examination). This book consists of a series of cases or clinical problems which will be broken into sections to help you deal with such a case, regardless of whether it is a long case, short case or a station in an OSCE. Each case will be given an indication of the likelihood of that type of case appearing in the exam. This can only be indicative, as certain conditions – for example thalassaemias – may only be seen commonly in larger metropolitan centres. There are five categories: very unlikely, unlikely, possible, likely and very likely. Categorization will apply to the type of case and also to the different possible diagnoses. For example, it may be very likely that you will be presented with a breathless child but only possible that you might see a case of bronchiolitis. Remember, some candidates may still meet cases which would be considered unlikely in the exam. View this as an opportunity to shine rather than terrible luck!

The likelihood will be indicated as follows:	
★	Very unlikely
★★	Unlikely
★★★	Possible
★★★★	Likely
★★★★★	Very likely

PREPARING FOR THE CLINICAL EXAMINATION

You have already met people who you know had absolutely every word in the standard textbooks off by heart, and frightened you over coffee by their apparent knowledge. These are sometimes the ones who say 'Oh I've not even begun to study yet', when you know they were up all last night memorizing stuff. Most of these people do obnoxiously well throughout medical school, but a proportion fall at the hurdle of clinical/oral examinations. One of their problems is that the questions asked are often not the type that can be answered by regurgitating a paragraph from a textbook. Usually you rely on being able to synthesize an answer from a variety of sources, the most important of which is your clinical experience. Candidates who have been around the wards learn as much by osmosis from those around them as they do from books.

Many of the elements of clinical and viva examinations resemble concert performances. It is useful to consider how a performer prepares. The first method is rehearsal. Clearly, adequate rehearsal includes a knowledge of the particular format of the exam that you are sitting. The techniques of answering questions in a long case and in short cases and OSCEs are quite different. Regardless of which format is being used, the value of mock exams cannot be overemphasized and you should attempt to rehearse for all possible scenarios. Notwithstanding rehearsal, on the day a performer should look the part.

Personal presentation

Do not be insulted if this is too obvious to you. Some candidates still present themselves as slovenly, and although you might not agree with your examiners' ideas of sartorial elegance you will influence their approach to you by your appearance. Conservative dress is the rule, with a dark suit, plain black shoes and a non-club tie. Women do not usually need to be given direction on how to present themselves, but the rule about suits is still a useful one.

Consider how you form impressions of people you never speak to. Even just sitting on the train or on a bus, you make assumptions about those around you. Whether those assumptions are in any way justified is exceedingly doubtful, but think about how readily you form them.

In a long case format exam it is likely that the first time the examiners see you will be when introduced by the invigilator. The examiners might introduce themselves, or even shake hands. Do not be taken aback by this show of humanity, but remember that they will already have formed an impression of you. Thus, for example, your stance is terribly important. You need not stand to attention, but certain postures imply a lack of respect for the examiners: leaning against a handy radiator with your legs crossed at the ankles is definitely to be avoided, as is folding your arms in the presence of the examiners. In body language terms this is definitely not to be recommended. The impression given by such a posture is that you are putting up barriers or resisting questions. Even if you think you never do this, ask your colleagues. Better still, if you can arrange a mock examination see if someone will videotape it for you. You will be amazed at how often you bring your hands to your ears or mouth, or adopt mannerisms of which you are unaware but which become pronounced under stress and which can annoy examiners.

In OSCEs you will be moving between stations and the examiners will remain seated at the station. Thus the onus is generally on the candidate to introduce himself or herself to the examiners or, if present, a mock patient, or both.

You should learn which posture you are comfortable in, both standing at the bedside and sitting at an OSCE station. Some candidates, for example, don't know what to do with their hands when being asked questions, and it is possible to become quite clumsy in such a situation. In either format you may have been given a clipboard with paper upon which to make notes. Keep this in your hands. This is helpful for two reasons: the first is that it allows you to refresh your memory occasionally, and the second is that it stops you scratching your nose or eyebrows, etc. Do not read from your notes as if you have a short-term memory defect – they are there to act as prompts, not as a script for your case history.

LONG CASES, SHORT CASES AND OSCES

Long cases

Some medical schools will examine students on a 'long case', which might come from any specialty. In other words, if the type of exam is a long case then the candidate may be presented with a psychiatric case, a pregnant woman or a man with a hernia, and may not know what type of case he or she will see until introduced to the patient. Others maintain the tradition of examination by specialty, i.e. medicine on Monday, surgery on Wednesday, etc. Regardless of which system prevails in your school, you will still need to approach the finals with a breadth of knowledge of all the key disciplines.

It is as well to remember that some poor registrar, with varying degrees of good grace, has been landed with the task of finding cases for the clinical part of the examination, and it is not always possible for him or her to find good cases.

You will be asked to present your case, and different examiners will expect different styles of presentation. Particular styles for each specialty are suggested in each section of this book, but to some extent it does not matter how you present your case as long as it is logical. Practise speaking much more slowly than you are accustomed to. Often candidates speak very rapidly indeed, and it can be difficult for examiners to identify that your perceptive, incisive comments are not just babble. This should be commented on by people helping you with mock cases.

A word on jargon

Medicine is bedevilled by jargon, and an ability to use this effectively is worth acquiring. Remember that the function of jargon is to communicate ideas efficiently, not to confuse patients or to set you apart by its exclusiveness. Remember also that some examiners object to excessive use of jargon and to some abbreviations: some consultants prefer to avoid terms such as CCF or COPD, but you should certainly be familiar with them and comfortable in their use.

Anticipating questions

The good candidate should be able to anticipate at least some of the more likely questions. For example, if in gynaecology you have presented a case of postmenopausal bleeding, it is sensible to anticipate a question such as 'What are the causes of postmenopausal bleeding?' or 'How should such a case be managed?'

Some points about answering questions in the clinical exam need some emphasis, and this relates to the appropriate use of words. For example, the staging of all malignancies has fixed definitions, but other conditions do not. You should know these and describe the value of staging and how it may help to plan management. If you use words like 'moderate' or 'early' disease, then you should have your mind made up about the answer to the question 'What do you mean by "moderate"?' Another awful word you may use is 'monitor', as in 'I will monitor disease progression'. What do you really mean by that? The actual phrase means virtually nothing. Thus in a case of MI it is better to say that you will measure the cardiac enzymes daily rather than 'monitor' them, because that is what the examiner wishes to know.

Another prevalent and annoying response from candidates is to repeat the question. There is almost nothing more infuriating for an examiner than to ask a question and have their words repeated to them. They may feel, subconsciously or otherwise, that the candidate is astonished at the apparent stupidity of the question, which offends them a little, or that the candidate is deaf. Neither approach is helpful in passing the examination. You may think you never do this, but check with other people and take note of how often other candidates do.

In long cases there is often an oral component to the exam which is held away from the patient and in which you may be asked anything about the discipline and, if you are unlucky, may be questioned on topics covered in your preclinical years, such as physiology or anatomy.

Slides and 'pots' may be presented to you for comment.

The layout of the cases described in this book usually begins with a definition, as a common starting question for any long case is: 'and what exactly do you mean by pre-eclampsia/ inflammatory bowel disease/dyspnoea/failure to thrive?' etc. There is a disappointing number of candidates who stand opened-mouthed for some moments in these circumstances in clinical and oral examinations. Rote learning is currently being discouraged in favour of 'problem-based learning'. Nevertheless, the inability to give a straightforward definition of a common clinical condition may well constitute an own goal – or is at least time wasting – and psychologically it is a bad way of introducing yourself to the examiners.

The next section for each case will usually relate to the relevant features you might either identify or exclude in the history. It is not the intention here to describe how to take a history: you should have sorted that out by now. It is intended to highlight for you the parts of the history which you should emphasize for the examiners.

Similarly, the clinical examination section serves to point out the particular findings of relevance in these cases. In addition to the long case, depending on the specialty and the medical school, you may also be presented with short cases which require that you identify specific clinical signs.

At the end of some sections on examination technique for individual cases is a section on 'facts'. These are intended as little 'tasters' so that you can go back to the textbooks and find out more. Remember, this is not a textbook, but it can nudge you into looking things up. Other facts are included just for general interest. Some of these items lend themselves to particular questions, and you might care to imagine which might be asked about in your examination.

Discussion points may follow and you might again consider which of these might reasonably be raised in the examination. They may be suited either to a discussion at the end of a long case or as specific points in short cases or OSCEs.

Short cases

Some aspects of the long case presentation may be very similar to those encountered in short cases. Essentially, however, short cases usually consist of clinical signs or aspects of history taking. Identifying clinical signs will lead to more in-depth discussion of the case. Generally, short cases allow both candidate and examiner to get to the fundamentals of the clinical problem, rather than assessing your history taking and presentation skills.

OSCEs

Increasingly, medical schools are using this type of exam to evaluate student performance. The background to this is that the conventional long and short cases which have previously been used, and are often still used, suffer from a degree of subjectivity on the part of the examiners. Furthermore, they lack consistency from candidate to candidate. Many students are familiar with the concept of the difficult patient and not all examiners are able to adjust appropriately for the underlying difficulty posed by the variability in clinical material. Thus, for example, for the candidate in a surgical finals, a woman who has a breast cancer but who has had a CVA and is dysphasic may present a greater challenge than a much younger woman presenting with a fibroadenoma, irrespective of the underlying pathology or clinical signs. OSCEs remove that subjectivity.

Most OSCEs comprise a number of different stations, usually with a similar time at each. The time interval ranges from 5 minutes to 20 minutes and varies between specialties and medical schools.

It is impossible to give an all-embracing breakdown of the different types of OSCE. The more common types of station are as follows:

- *Format 1: Standardized patient*   An actor following a standardized script would normally play this. An example would be to have a patient presenting with weight loss.
- *Format 2: Data recognition*   This could be an ECG or cardiac enzymes with a request for interpretation. These could be tied in with cases on chest pain.
- *Format 3: Communications station*   An example would be in the section on contraception where the candidate would be invited to discuss alternative methods with either an examiner or a standardized patient.
- *Format 4: Practical procedure*   An example might be: 'Examine the chest of this breathless man.' Alternatives could involve mannequins, for example: 'Perform a pelvic examination on this model.'
- *Format 5: Structured oral examination*   This usually follows the format of a question on a clinical topic followed by a number of preset questions. There is the potential for a more objective assessment by the examiner in this type of case.

In the first type of OSCE station, the standardized patient, the candidate is commonly presented with a person who has been given a script to 'act to'. Your task will vary; you may already have been given a short note along the lines of 'You are the receiving house physician and you are asked to see a 24-year-old woman with sudden onset of breathlessness.' From there you take a history focusing on this. Depending on how interactive the actor has been instructed to be, he or she may even interrupt you; for example, while you are taking your history a female actor might say something like 'Do you think my pill could be causing this Doctor?'

The second type, the data recognition type of station, is usually a straightforward series of questions accompanying the evidence. Thus, with an ECG your instructions might indicate that this tracing has been taken from an obese 53-year-old man with sudden onset of chest pain. The follow-up questions may be along the lines of 'What abnormalities do you see?', followed by 'What further investigations might you undertake?', and then by 'What treatment would you recommend?', and so on.

The communications station may also involve an actor, or the examiner may play the patient role. An example might be that you have been asked to obtain preoperative consent from a man about to undergo cholecystectomy. Generally you will be expected to cover a number of specifics; for example, the type of anaesthesia that will be used, the type of procedure, laparoscopic or open, duration of operation and recovery time, etc.

The practical skill type of station may involve a clinical sign; for example, you might be asked to take the pulse of a real patient with AF. This station is similar to a short case but may not need so much clinical detail. The function of such a station is to assess the examination technique rather than factual knowledge. There is increasing use of mannequins as teaching aids, and commonly in gynaecological cases you may be presented with an artificial pelvis and asked to 'take a smear'.

The structured oral type of station usually involves you answering a set of questions from the examiner, whose role is to identify whether your knowledge covers the specifics required for a given topic. There will usually be a key question to set the scene: 'What causes of hypertension are you familiar with?', followed by 'If we concentrate on renal causes, what conditions would you consider?', etc.

One of the key points about OSCEs is that every examiner should have the same marking scheme. Every candidate should be asked the same questions and the accepted answers are decided when the questions are set, not during the examination itself. Most of the cases in this handbook will include sections on how a particular case or clinical problem might be used in an OSCE.

Finally, do remember that, while being very fair and objective, OSCEs are astonishingly boring for the examiners, who might ask the same series of questions 20, 30 or more times in a day.

The impossible question

Inevitably there will be occasions when you are asked a question which you do not have a clue how to answer. There may be different reasons for this. Let us dispense with the possibility that it might be plain ignorance on your part. One problem is that examiners do sometimes ask questions that are obscure or ambiguous: there can be bad examiners as well as bad candidates. This is much more probable in a long case than a short case or OSCE. You should have a strategy for dealing with impossible questions: it is important that if you are asked about something you have not even heard of you should say so, in order to move on to something else. If you hum and haw, the examiners will assume you are ignorant of this obscure topic, so try to move on rapidly so as to leave them with an impression of knowledge rather than ignorance.

Another type of impossible question is one where you are not certain what the examiner is getting at. This is likely to be a management-type question rather than one of fact and, again, more likely in a long case than in an OSCE. There are three options in this situation. The first is to answer the question as well as you can understand it with as near as possible to a factual answer. Alternatively, if you really do not know what the examiner means, make a simple statement of fact relating to the general topic. With these approaches you will score points with factually correct comments that force the examiner to rephrase the question, hopefully in a better way. The third option is to make clear that you do not understand the question the way it is phrased. This requires tact, but in long cases there are usually two examiners and the other examiner may be grateful to you because he or she might not see what his or her colleague is getting at either! This is a final resort but immeasurably better than forcing the examiner to ask the question again because of an embarrassingly prolonged silence. A long silence is time wasted when you should be impressing the examiners.

In answering questions you should try to give all the relevant information you have been asked for. This can be likened to jumping a ravine: with your first answer you want to get right over to the other side. Some candidates leave the exam saying they have answered hundreds of questions, all of them correctly. What they do not realize is that their answers just get them to the crumbly edge at the other side, and every question they answer just keeps them there, without reaching solid ground. In these circumstances you occasionally find examiners of the 'Oh really, Doctor?' variety. These are the people who, after you have outlined a course of management or stated a fact, say something like 'Do you really think so?' Sometimes they are trying to make you change your mind, and sometimes will succeed so well that the candidate ends up condemning his or her original opinion. If you are confident that your original answer represented good practice, then you should be able to defend it, although you are at liberty to say that the question addresses a controversial subject.

MEDICINE

HISTORY AND EXAMINATION IN MEDICINE

The essence of history and examination in medicine is essentially the same for all disciplines; try to focus on the key elements of the history and examination, as these should be emphasized when presenting your findings to the examiner. Try to be concise with your presentation technique as this implies your ability to focus on what is important (and what is not!). Use appropriate medical terms when talking to the examiners: conventionality is expected and makes you 'look the part'.

Compare these two opening sentences: 'Mr A is a 62-year-old man complaining of shortness of breath. He has coughed up blood on two occasions. He is a smoker. His appetite is poor and he has lost some weight.' Alternatively, you could summarize this more elegantly: 'Mr A is a 62-year-old smoker presenting with dyspnoea, haemoptysis, anorexia and weight loss.' The same information is imparted but the second, more succinct technique has an air of authority and confidence which is likely to impress the examiner. It also immediately focuses the mind on a diagnosis of bronchial carcinoma until proven otherwise.

In the medical part of the final MBChB you are more likely to encounter multiple pathology, for example the patient with rheumatoid disease and ischaemic heart disease. This is especially so for long cases. In this eventuality you will need to adopt a more holistic approach, placing each disease in the context of the other. For example, the patient may not be suitable for exercise testing if mobility is significantly restricted. Equally, rheumatoid patients frequently have chronic anaemia, which may exacerbate anginal symptoms. You should think about such issues and be prepared to discuss them with the examiner. The management of most disease processes is influenced by comorbidity and you should be able to use a commonsense approach when asked about the further investigation and management of the patient on an individual basis. In medicine, patients often have debilitating diseases and you should take a detailed social history to determine the extent of social support which may be required to assist the patient with activities of daily living. If the examiners choose to discuss such issues you will obviously not require knowledge from a medical textbook – good common sense will suffice.

Finally, and inevitably, you will encounter the 'What are the causes of . . . ?' question. Equally inevitably, your mind may go blank. In this eventuality do not panic. Use the following mnemonic (DIVINE HATTI) as an *aide-mémoire* but remember that common things occur commonly.

Degenerative	**H**ereditary
Infective	**A**utoimmune
Vascular / Ischaemic	**T**raumatic
Iatrogenic (e.g. medication)	**T**oxins (e.g. alcohol)
Neoplastic	**I**diopathic
Endocrine	

THE CASES

CEREBROVASCULAR DISORDERS ★★★★★

Patients with cerebrovascular disease (CVA or TIA) are ideal long or short cases in final exams.

A patient with a good history of a TIA makes an ideal long case. Alternatively, you may be asked to perform a limited neurological examination at an OSCE station (e.g. examine the upper limbs or cranial nerves). You may be asked to communicate with a dysphasic patient.

DEFINITIONS

- **Transient ischaemic attack** Focal neurological deficit resulting from cerebral ischaemia which resolves completely within 24 hours.
- **Stroke** Focal neurological deficit due to a vascular lesion which persists for longer than 24 hours if the patient survives.

HISTORY

In a long case, as with any disease state, obtain an accurate history of the events. Which function(s) are impaired? How has the deficit worsened or improved? Were there any premonitory symptoms (approximately 25% report a prior TIA)? Was speech or understanding affected? Attention must also be directed to risk factors, e.g. smoking, family history, hypertension, diabetes, obesity and the oral contraceptive pill. Find out how many cigarettes are smoked, whether hypertension has been treated, etc. Also establish whether there is evidence of other vascular disease, e.g. myocardial ischaemia or peripheral vascular disease.

MEDICINE

EXAMINATION

The clinical diagnosis of a stroke is usually straightforward. Remember, however, that if signs of neurological deficit are persisting, then by definition you cannot diagnose a TIA.

In a long case, general examination should note evidence of hyperlipidaemia (e.g. corneal arcus in the young patient or xanthelasma), facial asymmetry, gaze paresis or typical hemiplegic posture. You should look for any source of emboli such as AF or carotid bruits. Measuring BP is mandatory, and if it is elevated, then examination of the fundi is indicated. Thereafter you should examine the central nervous system, including the cranial nerves.

As a short case or OSCE you may be expected to compare one side with the other. Look for evidence of homonymous hemianopia and facial weakness. Power, tone, reflexes and sensation should be assessed for all limbs. Remember to use reinforcement if reflexes are absent or difficult to initiate. Test for clonus. To avoid confusion when describing findings, it is often better to refer to left-sided weakness or hemiplegia, rather than right-sided CVA. This is the kind of statement that can start examiners asking about cerebrovascular anatomy and dominant hemispheres, etc.

FACTFILE

1. Know your reflexes: biceps C5/6
                                     supinator C5/6
                                     triceps C6/7
                                     knee L3/4
                                     ankle L5/S1.

2. Expressive (Broca's area – dominant frontoparietal lobes) and receptive dysphasia (Wernicke's area – dominant temporoparietal lobes) often coexist, although one may predominate. If you suspect expressive dysphasia, show the patient a pen and ask if it is a comb? The patient with expressive

---

dysphasia will answer 'No', whereas no meaningful reply will ensue from the patient with receptive dysphasia.

3. Clonus is rhythmical involuntary muscular contraction due to abrupt stretching. It is most easily detected at the ankle or knee joints and is indicative of an upper motor neurone problem.

4. Grade power in the limbs according to the following scale:
   0 No active contraction
   1 Visible or palpable contraction but no limb movement
   2 Movement possible when gravity eliminated
   3 Movement possible against gravity
   4 Movement possible against gravity and resistance but weaker than normal
   5 Normal power.

5. Reinforcement. Ask the patient to clench the teeth (upper limb reflexes) or to clench the hands and pull in opposite directions (lower limbs). Remember reinforcement only lasts about 1 second so the clenching manoeuvre must be performed simultaneously with the blow from the tendon hammer.

6. Dedicated stroke units which specialize in the management of cerebrovascular disease have been shown to improve patient outcome.

7. Swallowing should be assessed promptly after a stroke to avoid recurrent aspiration.

8. TIAs are an important prognostic event.

9. Within 5 years of a TIA, 1 out of 6 patients will have suffered a stroke.

10. Within 5 years of a TIA, 1 in 4 will die (usually from heart disease or stroke).

11. Approximately 80% of strokes are thromboembolic, whereas 20% arise from intracranial haemorrhage.

12. Within the first month, mortality from a thromboembolic CVA is less than 25%; approximately 75% with a haemorrhagic CVA will die.

Discussion points

1. Be prepared to discuss further investigation of stroke/ TIA. This is likely to include ECG, carotid Dopplers, echo and CT scanning.

2. Be prepared to discuss risk factor modification: treatment of hypertension, AF and cessation of smoking, etc.

3. Your patient communication skills could be tested here (e.g. 'Discuss life-style modification with this lady who suffered a stroke last week.').

4. Be able to discuss signs or symptoms with reference to the area of brain affected, e.g. parietal, cerebellar, frontal, etc.

5. Be familiar with early indicators of a poor prognosis after a stroke (e.g. coma, severe hemiplegia, gaze paresis).

6. Be able to draw the optic pathways and explain the anatomical basis of a hemianopia.

7. You may be asked about possible aids that patients may require to allow them to return home (e.g. stair lifts, shower instead of bath, commode).

THE DYSPNOEIC PATIENT ★★★★★

DEFINITION

Dyspnoea is a subjective awareness of difficulty breathing.

As dyspnoea is very common you are likely to encounter this complaint in an exam. There are many possible causes but most will be obvious from the history. The long case will test your ability to take a detailed history and draw up a plausible differential diagnosis. You can thereafter expect to be questioned on further investigation and management.

Most patients who complain of dyspnoea will also have physical signs that are ideal for a short case or OSCE station (e.g. 'Examine this lady's chest or heart.'). Alternatively, you may be asked to give instruction on how to use a salbutamol inhaler at a communication station.

The most likely causes of dyspnoea seen in an exam are:

- congestive cardiac failure ★★★★★★
- chronic obstructive pulmonary disease ★★★★★
- asthma ★★★★★
- pleural effusion ★★★★
- bronchial carcinoma ★★★★
- pneumonia ★★★★
- pneumothorax ★★★
- pulmonary thromboembolism ★★★
- pulmonary fibrosis ★★★
- bronchiectasis ★★★
- cystic fibrosis ★★★

HISTORY

Try to establish whether the cause of dyspnoea is cardiac or respiratory in origin (or both). Orthopnoea or paroxysmal nocturnal dyspnoea suggests a cardiac cause. A past medical history of MI, long-standing hypertension or rheumatic fever is relevant. A detailed smoking history is essential. Remember the six cardinal symptoms of respiratory disease: cough, sputum, haemoptysis, dyspnoea, wheeze, pain. In a patient with asthma, ask about nocturnal or exertional symptoms. A history of atopy should be sought. Exposure to industrial agents or household pets should be noted. **NB**: If you encounter a young patient with finger clubbing, dyspnoea and sputum production in the finals, he or she will almost certainly have cystic fibrosis. Establish the family history.

EXAMINATION

Remember to perform this in the standard manner: inspection, palpation, percussion and auscultation. You should be guided by history, but seek evidence of cardiovascular or respiratory disease. Look for clubbing, signs of anaemia and

MEDICINE

weight loss. Comment on respiratory rate and presence of cyanosis. Coexistent eczema in a young person with intermittent dyspnoea suggests asthma. Respiratory examination should note the hyperinflated chest of emphysema/COPD. Tracheal deviation is rarely detected but should be sought. Asymmetric chest expansion may reveal underlying lung pathology. If any abnormalities are detected, establish whether these are consistent with the patient's history. Cardiovascular examination should detect tachycardia, cardiomegaly, elevated JVP, peripheral oedema, cardiac murmurs and basal crepitations.

FACTFILE

1. **The following features suggest a severe attack of asthma:**
   (a) use of accessory muscles of respiration
   (b) inability to speak
   (c) severe tachycardia (or worse, bradycardia)
   (d) diminished breath sounds
   (e) cyanosis
   (f) normal or increased $P\text{CO}_2$ ($P\text{CO}_2$ usually decreases in asthma due to hyperventilation).

2. Pneumothorax should always be excluded in acute asthma.

3. The British Thoracic Society provide stepwise guidelines to the management of chronic asthma; these are due to be updated soon.
   Step 1 – Occasional use of relief bronchodilators
   Step 2 – Regular inhaled steroid plus short-acting inhaled beta agonists
   Step 3 – High-dose inhaled steroids plus short-acting beta agonists or low-dose inhaled steroids plus long-acting beta agonist (salmeterol)
   Step 4 – High-dose inhaled steroids plus regular bronchodilators
   Step 5 – Add regular oral steroids

4. Before moving up a step, inhaler technique should be checked and patient education should be reinforced. Poor inhaler technique is a common cause of failure to control symptoms.

5. Treatment should be reviewed every 3–6 months in the hope of stepping down.

6. Patients should be taught to monitor peak flow rates.

7. Spontaneous pneumothorax is more common in tall thin males and in patients with lung disease.

8. Staining of the fingers is caused by tar, not nicotine. This seems rather trivial, but is usually a source of amusement for the examiner.

9. Never settle for a diagnosis of CCF. Try to identify the cause, e.g. IHD or valvular heart disease.

10. A Scottish heart failure database revealed a 3-year mortality of 65%. Patients with severe heart failure symptoms (i.e. at rest) have a 50% mortality rate at 1 year.

11. In the treatment of CCF, diuretics should be used to relieve symptoms of fluid overload. Thereafter the lowest possible dose of diuretic should be used for maintenance, along with the highest tolerated dose of ACE inhibitor and beta blocker.

Discussion points

1. Know how to treat an acute episode of pulmonary oedema.
2. Know the management of an acute exacerbation of asthma.
3. Know the difference between a transudate and an exudate and the causes of each (see below).
4. Know the features of finger clubbing (loss of nailbed angle, increased curvature of the nail and fluctuation of the nailbed). Be prepared to discuss causes (see below) but remember common things occur commonly.
5. Be aware of the common causes of occupational lung disease in the UK.

6. Be prepared to discuss the investigation of bronchial carcinoma and assessment for possible surgical treatment.

Transudate (<30 g protein per litre)
- Cardiac failure
- Nephrotic syndrome
- Hepatic failure

Exudate (>30 g protein per litre)
- Pneumonia (including TB)
- Malignancy ($1°$ or $2°$)
- Pulmonary infarction
- Subphrenic abscess
- Meigs' syndrome (with ovarian fibroma)

Causes of finger clubbing
Respiratory ★★★★★
- Chronic suppurative lung disease (e.g. empyema, bronchiectasis, cystic fibrosis, abscess)
- Fibrosing alveolitis
- Bronchial carcinoma
- Mesothelioma

Cardiovascular
- Cyanotic congenital heart disease
- Infective endocarditis

Gastrointestinal ★★
- Cirrhosis
- Inflammatory bowel disease
- GI lymphoma

Others (rare) ★
- Familial
- Thyrotoxicosis

CHEST PAIN ★★★★★

Chest pain is one of the most common reasons for acute admission to hospital. It is therefore not surprising that it is also one of the most common conditions to be encountered in the final MB examination. A typical exam scenario would be a long case format with discussion of the case thereafter. In the exam the most likely causes of chest pain are:

- angina pectoris ★★★★★
- myocardial infarction ★★★★★
- pleuritic pain ★★★★
- pulmonary thromboembolus ★★★
- pneumothorax ★★★
- oesophageal pain ★★

DEFINITIONS

- **Angina pectoris** Literally means pain in the chest, assumed to be due to ischaemia of the myocardium.
- **Myocardial infarction** Arises when necrosis of the cardiac muscle occurs.
- **Pneumonia** Inflammation of the lung, usually arising from bacterial or viral infection.
- **Pulmonary embolism** A condition arising from the passage of thrombus from the systemic veins or, occasionally, the right heart to the pulmonary arteries, resulting in pulmonary infarction and occasionally acute right ventricular failure.
- **Pneumothorax** Air in the pleural space.

HISTORY

The important features of cardiac pain are the relationship to exertion, the radiation to arm, jaw or neck and the character of the pain, which is classically crushing and central. The use of a clenched fist to describe the pain is highly suggestive of a cardiac origin (Levine's sign). Patients who describe a stabbing pain or point with one finger to the source of pain are unlikely to be experiencing myocardial ischaemia. The typical risk factors of family history, smoking, diabetes, hypertension, previous MI and elevated cholesterol should be noted.

Pleuritic pain is usually well described by patients. Associated dyspnoea is almost universal. Dyspnoea with associated collapse suggests a large pulmonary embolus (even in the absence of pleuritic pain). The production of sputum, haemoptysis or fever may suggest an infective origin. Coexistent calf pain or predisposing factors for DVT should be sought. In women ask about oral contraceptive usage. In young asthenic males with pleuritic pain, a pneumothorax is highly likely. A history of chest wall trauma is obviously relevant.

Oesophageal pain is notoriously difficult to differentiate from pain of cardiac origin. In addition, oesophageal and cardiac pathology often coexist. Previous investigation, such as barium meal or upper GI endoscopy with definite evidence of hiatus hernia or reflux oesophagitis, is worthy of note. Symptoms of 'heartburn' that are worse when bending over or recumbent suggest a possible oesophageal origin, although don't forget that decubitus angina is a recognized phenomenon.

EXAMINATION

Examination in ischaemic heart disease is frequently unhelpful. Look for signs of anaemia or thyrotoxicosis, which may precipitate or worsen the ischaemic symptoms. Xanthelasma or xanthomata should be noted. Occasionally there may be a cardiac murmur of relevance (e.g. aortic stenosis). Evidence of cardiac failure post-MI is relevant prognostically. In patients with pleuritic chest pain, look for asymmetry of chest wall expansion and comment on whether the patient is tachypnoeic or breathless. The presence of fever, anaemia, finger clubbing or emaciation should not be overlooked. If a sputum pot is present beside the bed, you must look at the contents. Do not forget to look for evidence of DVT.

FACTFILE

1. AMI is the most common cause of death in the UK.

2. In the UK Heart Attack Study, overall case fatality was 44%. Of those who died, 75% did so before admission to hospital, mostly as a result of ventricular fibrillation.

3. The cause of AMI is thrombus formation on an atherosclerotic plaque in a coronary artery.

4. Aspirin reduces mortality in AMI by ~25%.

5. Thrombolytic therapy reduces mortality in ST elevation AMI by approximately 25%. The benefits are additive to those of aspirin.

6. Thrombolytic therapy is indicated for patients with acute ST elevation or LBBB on their ECG. Patients with ST depression, T wave inversion and a normal ECG should not receive thrombolysis.

7. Thrombolytic therapy is more efficacious with earlier administration. Door-to-needle times in emergency departments must therefore be minimized and should be less than 30 minutes.

8. In addition to aspirin and thrombolytics, beta blockers, statins and ACE inhibitors have also been shown to reduce mortality following AMI.

9. Life-style measures must be addressed following AMI. Smoking cessation is the greatest single intervention in reducing the risk of further infarction.

10. The average cholesterol level in the UK is ~6 mmol/l. Following myocardial infarction, statins should be prescribed to reduce the serum cholesterol by 30% or to below 5.0 mmol/l.

11. ACE inhibitors are indicated in people who develop LVF in association with AMI and in those with impaired LV function on echo.

12. In unstable angina and non-ST elevation MI, patients at high risk should be considered for early revascularization by means of coronary artery angioplasty/stenting or bypass surgery.

13. High-risk features in unstable angina include troponin rise, LV dysfunction, haemodynamic instability and recurrent pain despite antianginal medications.

Discussion points

1. Be prepared to discuss the complications of AMI and the role of secondary prevention/risk factor modification.

2. The role of exercise tolerance testing in the management of patients with ischaemic heart disease is important and may be discussed.

3. Be aware of the absolute and relative contraindications to thrombolytic therapy.

4. Know the management of tension pneumothorax and the conditions associated with pneumothorax (i.e. virtually any respiratory disease).

5. Be prepared to discuss the possible causes of a pneumonia not responding to antibiotic therapy, e.g. atypical pneumonia, underlying neoplasm, TB, etc.

FINGER ON THE PULSE ★★★★★

On at least one occasion during your final examination in medicine you will have to examine and report the pulse. This may be as part of a modified short case or as an OSCE station. This should be a simple task, but the following points are worthy of note. You should comment on:

- rate
- rhythm
- character
- volume.

If you can perform this quickly and accurately you may impress by offering to check for radiofemoral delay and to listen for bruit (e.g. carotids).

RATE

Give an exact figure, never say approximately. You will have counted the pulse accurately and therefore it is entirely inappropriate to say 'approximately 78 per minute'. Bradycardia is defined as a heart rate below 60 beats/min. The most likely cause in an examination would be beta blocker therapy. Other possible causes are a previously athletic individual, or hypothyroid patients. Tachycardia is a heart rate >100 beats/min. Common causes are pyrexia, cardiac failure, exercise, anaemia and anxiety (compare with your own).

RHYTHM

If the rhythm is completely regular, then say that it is sinus rhythm. If the pulse is irregular in rhythm and volume, the diagnosis is almost certainly AF. In the long case, record both apical and radial rates. If merely asked to examine the pulse in a short case, you will impress if you also offer to measure the apical rate. Remember, in atrial fibrillation the rate you report is the ventricular rate, e.g. 'The rhythm is atrial fibrillation, with a poorly controlled ventricular rate of 110 beats per minute.'

If the rhythm is basically regular with occasional extra added beats, this is likely to be an ectopic beat. As the ectopic beat arises early, the pulse volume will be low due to incomplete LV filling. (Very early ectopics can be impalpable at the radial artery.)

CHARACTER

If asked to examine the pulse, always raise the arm to check for a collapsing pulse, indicative of aortic incompetence or, very occasionally, patent ductus arteriosus (look out for

MEDICINE

flying pigs!). A plateau pulse (slow rising) indicates aortic stenosis. Pulsus alternans is alternating low volume and high volume beats which occur in severe LV failure. Pulsus paradoxus is an exaggeration of the physiological normal whereby pulse volume reduces on inspiration. You will never see this in an exam setting as it occurs in cardiac tamponade and in a severe acute asthmatic attack.

VOLUME

Avoid using terms such as 'strong' or 'weak' to describe the pulse. It is best to describe the volume as low, normal or high. Pulse volume reflects left ventricular stroke volume.

FACTFILE

1. A high volume pulse is observed in anaemia, carbon dioxide retention and sepsis.
2. A low volume pulse is seen in CCF and hypovolaemia.
3. The following are the most common causes of atrial fibrillation (not necessarily in order):
   - ischaemic heart disease
   - mitral valve disease
   - congestive cardiac failure
   - hypertension
   - alcohol (acute or chronic)
   - thyrotoxicosis.
4. In the over 65-year-old population, 5–10% of patients have AF.
5. The risk of stroke in non-rheumatic AF is approximately 5% per year.
6. The thromboembolic risk of rheumatic AF is in excess of 20% per year.
7. A history of a previous CVA or MI, hypertension, LVH and diabetes are predictive of a higher thromboembolic risk in patients with AF.
8. In randomized trials, warfarin reduced the risk of stroke by ~60% and aspirin by ~20%.

Discussion points

1. This is likely to include the possible causes of AF.
2. Be prepared to discuss the role of anticoagulant therapy in AF.
3. Be prepared to discuss the pharmacological treatment of AF.

THE CARDIAC MURMUR ★★★★★

DEFINITIONS

- **Murmur**   Turbulent blood flow within the heart which can be heard with the stethoscope.
- **Thrill**   A palpable murmur.
- **Apex beat**   The most inferolateral point on the chest wall where the apical impulse is palpable (usually in the 5th intercostal space and in the midclavicular line).
- **Heave**   A diffuse or forceful palpable impulse.

It is almost inevitable that you will be asked to examine the heart in an OSCE station. Undergraduates usually experience greatest anxiety and heartache when asked to perform cardiac auscultation. You may be asked to examine the 'cardiovascular system', 'precordium' or 'heart' and confusion can arise. In the final MB examiners will usually direct you clearly and may tell you to omit certain parts of the examination due to time constraints. Do not fret about this but, if you are uncertain, use the standard principle of inspection, palpation and auscultation (perform cardiac percussion at your peril). The inspection process is not dependent on the instruction and should be carried out similarly for all three instructions. If asked to examine 'the cardiovascular system' you should feel the pulse, check the JVP and offer to measure BP and listen to the bases. Examining 'the precordium' or 'the heart' should include the above but you may wish to clarify with the examiner whether he or she wishes you formally to examine the pulse. If asked to 'listen to the heart', proceed as for 'examine the heart'. You can justify your actions by saying that you wish to correlate your auscultatory findings with those of inspection and palpation. It is important to remember that you are not expected to identify every cardiac lesion but you should be able to time the murmur, describe where it is best heard and where it radiates to. You are far more likely to impress by performing a thorough, confident examination than the candidate who correctly diagnoses a 'full house' of cardiac murmurs but does so using poor technique. Do not worry about grading the murmur (3/6, etc.): it is more important to give a good description and suggest the most likely lesion. Remember that some murmurs may be equally loud throughout the precordium (and indeed may radiate widely) so you may be unable to distinguish between, for example, aortic stenosis and mitral incompetence. If this happens, do not panic. Describe your findings fully and be prepared to admit your uncertainty, offering a logical differential diagnosis.

HISTORY

You will not generally be asked to take a history in a short OSCE station. You are likely to be given a brief history, e.g. 'This lady complains of dyspnoea on exertion; please examine her heart.'

EXAMINATION

Sit the patient at 45° and then proceed as follows.

Inspection

Is the patient breathless or tachypnoeic? Is he or she cyanosed or anaemic? Are there any surgical scars? A left thoracotomy scar is indicative of previous mitral surgery for mitral stenosis. Look under the left breast in women. Is there a malar flush of mitral stenosis? Is there an audible click from a prosthetic valve? Is the JVP elevated?

Palpation

1. Feel for the apex beat (definition above). Make sure you can count intercostal spaces!
2. Is the apex beat displaced (LV dilatation), thrusting (LV hypertrophy), tapping (mitral stenosis) or is there a double apical impulse (dyskinetic segment)?
3. Is there a right ventricular heave (felt with the palm of the hand at the left parasternal area on expiration)?
4. Are there any thrills (feels like a cat purring)?

Auscultation

1. Listen firstly with diaphragm at the apex, lower left sternal edge, aortic and pulmonary areas.
2. Concentrate initially on the heart sounds. Can you hear them both? Is one of them abnormally loud? Are there additional heart sounds (3rd or 4th)?
3. Are there any murmurs? If so, are they systolic or diastolic? Is it heard in any particular area or throughout the precordium. Is it high or low pitched?
4. Listen for radiation to both sides of the neck (?aortic stenosis but beware carotid bruits).
5. Sit the patient forward and listen at the lower left sternal edge in expiration (?aortic incompetence). Listen for the absence of silence in diastole.
6. Listen with the bell at the mitral area and turn the patient on to the left side. Mitral stenosis is a low pitched rumble (hence the bell) in diastole.

Tips

- Always sit the patient at 45°.
- Always feel the carotid pulse during auscultation.
- Always roll the patient on to the left to listen for mitral lesions.

- Always listen in the neck.
- Always sit patients forward and ask them to hold their breath in expiration. Listen for the absence of complete silence during diastole – if aortic incompetence is present you will invariably hear it.
- Practice is vital – do it often and always follow the same technique until you can perform it automatically, even in the most stressful situations.
- If uncertain whether a murmur is systolic or diastolic remember this moderately insulting but generally fair observation: if the undergraduate can hear it easily it must be systolic.
- When asked to report your findings, adopt a structured response. Mention the apex beat, then thrills and heaves; thereafter report the heart sounds, and finally any murmurs. For example: 'The apex beat is displaced. There is an RV heave. Heart sound 2 is loud in the pulmonary position with a pansystolic murmur heard throughout the precordium but loudest at the apex and axilla.' Then think logically how you can tie these findings together: 'This would be consistent with LV dilatation secondary to mitral incompetence with resultant pulmonary hypertension and RV hypertrophy.'

FACTFILE

1. Causes of an impalpable apex beat: obesity, not feeling sufficiently laterally, emphysema, pericardial/pleural effusion and dextrocardia (very rare, but less so in exams).
2. A right ventricular heave arises from RV hypertrophy. This occurs in conditions that cause raised pressure in the right side of the heart.
3. The first heart sound arises from closure of the mitral and tricuspid valves. It is loud in mitral stenosis.

4. The second heart sound arises from closure of the aortic and pulmonary valves. A loud A2 or P2 occurs in systemic or pulmonary hypertension, respectively. A split second sound is normal in young people or may be due to an atrial septal defect or pulmonary stenosis. A2 may be quiet in aortic stenosis.

5. A third heart sound is normal in young people but also occurs in LV or RV failure.

6. A fourth heart sound occurs when the atria contract against a stiff ventricle, such as in the presence of LVH.

7. Mitral stenosis is becoming less common in the developed world. It occurs secondary to rheumatic fever.

8. Definitive treatment of mitral stenosis may require valve replacement but certain patients may be suitable candidates for percutaneous balloon mitral valvuloplasty.

9. Aortic stenosis is common, particularly in older patients. The most common cause is calcific degeneration but aortic stenosis also occurs secondary to congenital bicuspid valves (M > F).

10. Exertional pain, dyspnoea and syncope are the most frequent symptoms of aortic stenosis. Syncope on exertion is particularly ominous and may be a forerunner of sudden death.

11. Once symptoms arise from aortic stenosis, the prognosis is poor and valve replacement should be considered.

12. Patients with valvular lesions should be advised on the need for good dental hygiene and antibiotic prophylaxis when undergoing infection-prone procedures.

13. Echocardiography is the definitive investigation of cardiac murmurs.

14. Infective endocarditis is more likely to occur in valve lesions where there is a high velocity jet. It is therefore unlikely to occur in pure mitral stenosis and is more common in mitral incompetence.

Discussion points

1. This will usually focus on the causes of the various valve lesions.
2. Know some causes of pulmonary hypertension/RV hypertrophy.
3. How would you confirm a case of suspected infective endocarditis?

DIABETES MELLITUS ★★★★★

You are very likely to meet a diabetic in your finals. A diabetic with complications such as neuropathy or retinopathy forms a good long case candidate. The examiners will have plenty scope for interrogation on the management of blood glucose and the numerous vascular complications. Equally, OSCE stations may be encountered. Examples would be a communications station in which you are instructed to give advice on life-style changes to a newly diagnosed diabetic, or a data recognition station with a photograph of diabetic retinopathy on which you will be invited to comment.

DEFINITION

A state of hyperglycaemia arising from insufficient or ineffective endogenous insulin.

The diagnosis is based on either:

- symptoms of hyperglycaemia (know these) plus one diagnostic test, or
- two diagnostic tests in the absence of symptoms.

There are three diagnostic tests:

1. fasting blood glucose >6.0 mmol/l
2. random blood glucose >11.1 mmol/l
3. oral glucose tolerance test (see below).

The oral glucose tolerance test

The patient is fasted overnight then given a 75 mg glucose drink. Plasma glucose levels (mmol/l) are checked before and at 2 hours after ingestion.

Time	Normal	Impaired glucose tolerance (IGT)	DM
Pre	<6.0		>7.0
2 Hours	<7.8	7.8–11.1	>11.1

Type I DM (juvenile or insulin-dependent DM)

Presents in younger age group. Always requires insulin as there is insulin deficiency.

Type II DM (non-insulin-dependent or maturity-onset DM)

Adult-onset (usually >40 years). Prevalence increases with age but it is becoming more common in younger populations and has even been reported in teenagers. It is associated with obesity and carries a high cardiovascular risk. Type II DM is caused by a reduction in insulin secretion and insulin resistance.

HISTORY

Important points in the history are: symptoms of hyperglycaemia, i.e. polyuria, polydypsia and weight loss. Past medical history of diabetic emergencies should be noted. The presenting feature of diabetes may be one of the complications, e.g. arterial disease, retinopathy, neuropathy, skin infections, renal disease and autonomic neuropathy (diarrhoea, impotence). Establish how long the patient has been diabetic and what treatment is currently being used. Bear in mind that older patients may have unknowingly been diabetic for some time. Take a dietary history and establish whether blood or urine monitoring is performed at home. You should always ask about cardiovascular risk factors.

EXAMINATION

In a long case this may be directed by the history. You should assess skin condition, insulin injection sites and all pulses. Blood pressure must be recorded. Neurological examination should establish the presence or absence of reflexes and of sensory deficit (light touch and vibration sense). Examination of the eyes should be performed with dilated pupils – remember cataracts are more common in diabetics. If a urine sample is available, test for both glucose and protein.

In a short case or OSCE you will be directed to a specific area for examination.

FACTFILE

1. There are over one million cases in the UK, with probably the same number undiagnosed.
2. The incidence of type II DM is rising in parallel with the inexorable rise in obesity.
3. Diabetics die on average a decade earlier than non-diabetics, the majority from CVS causes.
4. The aim of treatment in both forms of diabetes is normo-glycaemia without causing hypoglycaemia.
5. Hypoglycaemia causes autonomic symptoms (sweating, tremor, hunger and nausea) and neuroglycopenic symp-toms (drowsiness, altered behaviour and reduced consciousness).

6. The cornerstone of treatment in DM is life-style modification – its importance cannot be overstressed.

7. Basic dietary point: take unrefined carbohydrates (potatoes, pasta, cereals) instead of refined carbohydrates (Pepsi and Mars bars).

8. To prevent MI and CVA, rigorous BP control is required in type II DM. BP targets are lower in diabetics than in their non-diabetic counterparts (diastolic 80 mmHg versus 85 mmHg).

9. ACE inhibitors and angiotensin II antagonists appear to have renoprotective effects over and above their antihypertensive effects.

10. Patients on insulin should perform home blood glucose monitoring and keep a diary of readings.

11. Microvascular complications are peculiar to diabetics. Disease in the small arteries in the retina, renal glomerulus and nerve sheaths are of special concern. Microvascular complications typically arise 10–20 years after diagnosis in younger patients and present earlier in older individuals.

12. Diabetes confers an excess risk of macrovascular disease. Stroke is increased twofold, MI three- to fivefold and amputation is 50 times more likely.

13. Diabetic women lose their premenopausal protection from CVS events.

14. Statins have proven clinical benefits in diabetics, even in those with no previous CVS history.

15. 'Brittle' diabetes has no strict definition but is usually reserved for patients who require frequent hospitalization for hypoglycaemia and/or ketoacidosis. It is wrong to blame the patient for this but it is true to say that most of these individuals are at least partly responsible; for example, many ignore life-style advice.

Discussion points

1. Know the treatment of diabetic emergencies.
2. Be prepared to discuss different insulin regimens.
3. Further discussions are likely to involve diabetic complications and their prevention.
4. Occasionally you may need to discuss the pharmacology of oral hypoglycaemic agents.
5. You may be asked to discuss how we can prevent the increase in obesity and type II DM.

JAUNDICE ★★★★★

DEFINITION

A yellow discoloration of the skin and sclerae due to an elevated serum bilirubin.

You may encounter a jaundiced patient in the medical or surgical final exams. This can be categorized in different ways and it is worthwhile learning a classification system. For the purposes of final examinations the following causes should be considered:

- cirrhosis   ★★★★★
- viral hepatitis   ★★★
- hepatic malignancy   ★★
  (primary or secondary)
- gallstones
- carcinoma of the pancreas   (see p. 90)
- carcinoma of the bile duct

Rarer causes are:

- haemolytic jaundice (e.g. haemoglobinopathy)   ★
- congenital hyperbilirubinaemia (e.g. Gilbert's
  syndrome)   ★

HISTORY

In long cases you should determine the duration of illness and whether or not it is progressive. Bear in mind the age of the patient. Older people with weight loss are likely to have malignancy, whereas young patients are more likely to have hepatitis. Pruritus, stool and urine colour will suggest if there is an obstructive component to the jaundice. An infective cause is suggested by a recent community or family outbreak or recent travel abroad (hepatitis A). Intravenous drug abuse, tattoos, homosexuality or recent transfusion may lead to hepatitis B or C. Farm workers, sewage workers and those who participate in water sports may contract leptospirosis. Ask about alcohol ingestion and any medication. Women with jaundice and pruritus may have primary biliary cirrhosis. A family history of recurrent jaundice suggests Gilbert's syndrome in Caucasians or haemoglobinopathy in Asians or Africans. Abdominal pain may be secondary to gallstones or is sometimes due to hepatomegaly.

In a short case you may be presented with a clinical sign, e.g. hepatomegaly, and simply asked to demonstrate it. In an OSCE situation an example may be of data interpretation in which you are shown a set of liver function tests and asked to interpret them. You may be asked what further investigations you would wish to undertake.

EXAMINATION

Look for the signs of chronic liver disease (spider naevi, palmar erythema, flapping tremor, leuconychia, etc.). If hepatomegaly is detected, describe the features (i.e. smooth, firm, regular, irregular, pulsatile, etc.). A knobbly, irregular liver suggests metastases. Splenomegaly is usually taken as evidence of portal hypertension. Look for ascites, which is common in cirrhosis. If urine is available, test it.

FACTFILE

1. Liver function tests will help differentiate posthepatic (obstructive) from hepatic jaundice.

2. Chronic hepatitis is defined as any hepatitis lasting 6 months or longer.

3. Cirrhosis is a histological diagnosis: it can be defined as a condition involving the entire liver, with necrosis of hepatocytes followed by fibrosis and nodule formation. These changes are irreversible.

4. Approximately two-thirds of patients with cirrhosis will develop gastro-oesophageal varices, of which approximately one-third will bleed.

5. The following features are poor prognostic indicators in cirrhosis:
   - hypoalbuminaemia
   - hyponatraemia
   - coagulopathy
   - ascites
   - persistent jaundice
   - continued alcohol ingestion
   - neuropsychiatric complications.

6. Hepatocellular carcinoma is a primary hepatic malignancy which is associated with a raised alpha-fetoprotein. Approximately 80% of cases occur in cirrhotic livers.

Discussion points

1. As in an OSCE station, you should recognize a cholestatic or hepatocellular picture when shown abnormal LFTs.
2. Have a structured scheme for the investigation of jaundice.
3. What is the cause of pruritus in obstructive jaundice?
4. Be prepared to discuss the management of bleeding oesophageal varices.

5. Know how to treat hepatic encephalopathy and the pre-cipitating factors.
6. Which malignant processes commonly metastasize to the liver?
7. Know which drugs cause hepatotoxicity.
8. Know the anatomical landmarks of the spleen and how clinically to differentiate splenomegaly from an enlarged kidney.

HYPERTENSION ★★★★

Occasionally in the finals you may encounter a patient who has been admitted for investigation and/or treatment of hypertension, or indeed following admission with one of its complications. If seen as a long case, you should try to assess the overall cardiovascular risk and determine whether there is evidence of end-organ damage. You should also pursue the possibility of secondary hypertension. Alternatively, you may be asked to demonstrate how you would measure a patient's BP as part of a practical procedure short OSCE station. It is hard to define what is an abnormally high BP but the British Hypertension Society have issued guidelines on the threshold for intervention, depending on the esti-mated CVS risk. More than 90% of cases of hypertension have no single cause (i.e. essential hypertension). In the exam, however, you are probably more likely to encounter secondary causes of hypertension.

Causes of systemic hypertension
1. Essential >90%   ★★★★★
2. Secondary causes   ★★★
    (a) Renal disease (esp. renovascular)
    (b) Endocrine disorders:
        Cushing's
        Conn's

phaeochromocytoma
acromegaly
(c) Coarctation of the aorta ★
(d) Pregnancy ★
(e) Drugs: ★★ oral contraceptives and corticosteroids are the most common.

HISTORY

Enquire how long the patient has been hypertensive and whether he or she has received treatment. Ask about risk factors such as alcohol, smoking, exercise, diet (including salt and fat) and diabetes. Determine if there is a previous history of cardiovascular or renal disease. Drug (including compliance) and family history are noteworthy. Hypertension is usually asymptomatic but at higher levels may occasionally cause headache. If headache is associated with palpitations, tremor, flushing or sweating, a phaeochromocytoma should be suspected. This is rare even in the finals.

EXAMINATION

In most patients the only sign will be the high BP. Check BP in both arms and, if time allows, recheck after a further 5 minutes. Feel all pulses, especially radial and femorals. Cardiac examination may reveal an apical heave and loud aortic second sound. Listen for abdominal, carotid and femoral bruit. Fundoscopy is essential. Always look for any pointer to a secondary cause, e.g. cushingoid features, acromegaly, enlarged polycystic kidneys.

Tips for measuring BP in an OSCE station
1. Seat the patient with the arm resting on a table (i.e. at the level of the heart).
2. Expose the arm (no clothing under the cuff).
3. Choose the right size of cuff (too small a cuff will give a higher reading).

MEDICINE

4. Feel the brachial pulse and inflate the cuff until the pulse is lost.
5. Deflate the cuff slowly with the mercury column at eye level.
6. Record the diastolic pressure at phase V (absence of sounds).
7. Check BP in the other arm now (the examiner will stop you if there are time pressures).
8. Above all, make sure you have practised this and are familiar with applying the cuff. If you haven't done it before this will be obvious to the patient/subject (let alone the examiner).

FACTFILE

1. Management of hypertension must firstly address life-style issues such as smoking, alcohol and salt intake, weight reduction and exercise. Weight reduction of 7 kg translates to a 12 mmHg reduction in BP.
2. The mortality and morbidity risk increases as BP increases.
3. Improved BP control has been shown to reduce the incidence of MI and to reduce both incidence of and mortality from CVA.
4. Secondary hypertension should be considered if age <35, hypokalaemia (not on diuretics) or resistant to therapy.
5. The presence of LVH on the ECG represents end-organ damage and a significant mortality risk. LVH can regress following improved BP control.
6. 'Routine' investigations should include urinalysis, U+Es, cholesterol, blood glucose and ECG to assess for target organ damage.
7. A 5–6 mmHg reduction in diastolic BP reduces the risk of stroke by 42% and CHD events by 14%.
8. The recommended BP target for hypertensives is 140/85. In diabetics, where tight BP control is crucial, the target is 140/80.

Discussion points

1. This will usually centre on risk factor modification.
2. Be prepared to discuss the pharmacology and side-effects of antihypertensive drugs.
3. What are the secondary causes of hypertension?

SORE JOINTS ★★★★

Arthritis is inflammation of the joint(s). The main types of arthritis are:

- rheumatoid arthritis   ★★★★★
- osteoarthritis   ★★★
- connective tissue disorders (e.g. SLE and systemic sclerosis)   ★★★
- ankylosing spondylitis   ★★★
- psoriatic arthritis   ★★★
- infective arthritis   ★★
- gout   ★★
- reactive arthritis   ★★

HISTORY

Establish which joint(s) are most affected, what time of day they are most sore and what degree of disability is present. How does the disability affect activities of daily living (e.g. dressing, washing, etc.) Is there a past medical history of trauma to the joint, or is there extra-articular involvement (e.g. lungs, eyes, skin)? Is there a family history of similar illness? Is there a history of autoimmune disease?

EXAMINATION

Examination of sore joints alone will usually be as part of a short case or OSCE station. Inspection is key. Look for the cardinal signs of inflammation: heat, swelling, tenderness and redness. Observe the patient moving the joints and always ask the patient if the joints are sore before touching them (inflicting pain on a patient immediately puts you on probation!). Does the patient appear anaemic? The classical rheumatoid changes, if present, should be obvious. Don't forget to look for rheumatoid nodules, a sign of seropositive RA. If possible, test the patient's ability to use a pen, cutlery, comb, etc. Look for evidence of muscle wasting and extra-articular involvement, e.g. scleritis, vasculitis, rashes (SLE, psoriasis).

FACTFILE

1. Early RA causes pain, stiffness and swelling in the joints, typically worse in the morning or after inactivity. Small joints (hands and feet) are typically affected and will be tender with swelling. Some patients will describe flu-like symptoms.

2. Indicators of a poorer prognosis in early RA are:
   multiple joint involvement
   high inflammatory parameters (ESR or CRP) at outset
   positive rheumatoid factor
   early X-ray changes
   poorer functioning at outset
   adverse socioeconomic circumstances and lower educational level.

3. Guidelines suggest that RA should be treated at an early stage with disease-modifying antirheumatic drugs (DMARDs), which can reduce symptoms and delay disease progression.

4. X-rays of rheumatoid joints will typically show soft tissue swelling, juxta-articular osteoporosis, loss of joint space, bony erosions and subluxation.

5. Swan neck deformity arises from hyperextension of the PIP and flexion of the DIP.

6. Boutonniere deformity has flexion at the PIP joint with a hyperextended PIP joint.

7. Rheumatoid arthritis is a common illness afflicting approximately 2% of the world population. Because of its systemic nature, rheumatoid disease is an appropriate term.

8. General anaesthesia (with endotracheal intubation) may be contraindicated in patients with RA because of cervical spine involvement. This is important because many rheumatoid patients may require joint replacement.

9. Aspirin and diuretics can increase serum urate and, if possible, should be avoided in patients with gout.

10. Allopurinol can prevent acute flare-ups but should not be commenced until the acute attack has settled.

Discussion points

1. Be prepared to discuss how RA may affect the patient's ability to perform everyday tasks, especially personal hygiene.

2. Know which drugs can be used as suppressive agents in the treatment of RA and what the side-effects are.

3. Be prepared to discuss the extra-articular features of RA and other connective tissue diseases.

4. What are the side-effects of NSAIDs?

FUNDOSCOPY ★★★★

Usually a component of a short case or OSCE, you should anticipate performing ophthalmoscopy in your final exams. This may spark panic in the reader but there is no need for alarm. The undergraduate is not expected to be an expert in diagnosing fundal abnormalities but you should be competent at performing the examination; you may even be asked to examine an actor with a normal fundus. Make sure you look familiar with the ophthalmoscope and know the principles behind the examination. In reality, there are very few fundal conditions that you are likely to encounter. These include:

- diabetic retinopathy ★★★★★
- hypertensive retinopathy ★★★★
- papilloedema ★★★★
- optic atrophy ★★★
- cataracts ★★★
- retinitis pigmentosa ★★★

HISTORY

You are unlikely to be asked to take any history but you may get the chance to ask a couple of questions. You may wish to ask if the patient/subject has had eye-drops instilled (pupillary reflexes may be lost). Ask if the patient has noticed a problem in one or both eyes. If the problem is uni-lateral, examine the 'normal' eye first. As in cardiac auscul-tation, develop a routine for ophthalmoscopy and stick with this. The following is suggested.

EXAMINATION

1. The environment should be suitably dark. If obviously not possible (e.g. the exam is in an open ward), then mention that ideally this should be the case. Explain to the patient/actor what you are going to do.
2. Take off spectacles (if appropriate).
3. Examine the right eye with your right eye and the scope in your right hand. Similarly, the left eye should be exam-ined with your left eye and the scope in your left hand. Ask the patient to fix the gaze on a distant object. Blink-ing is allowed but ask the patient not to look into the light unless specifically requested to do so.
4. From a distance of about 25 cm shine the light on the eye and check if the red reflex is present. A cataract is the most

likely interruption of the red reflex you will see in the exam.

5. While still looking through the scope, bring the head and scope close to the patient's eye, without touching it. Focus on the fundus, using corrective lenses as required for a clear view.

6. Examine the optic disc first.

7. Thereafter turn your attention to the arteries and veins. Follow the vessels out from the disc to each quadrant in turn.

8. Now look at the background, assessing each quadrant in turn.

9. Finally, ask the patient to look into the light. This brings the macula into view. It appears as a darker red patch on the temporal side of the fundus.

FACTFILE

1. Hard exudates are lipid-rich deposits.
2. Soft exudates are associated with retinal ischaemia or infarction.
3. Fundal abnormalities to look for at each site are as follows:
   (a) *Interruption of red reflex*
      - Opacities of lens, cornea or vitreous (cataract is the most likely exam abnormality).
   (b) *Optic disc*
      - Pallor, much whiter than expected (optic atrophy).
      - Papilloedema (swelling of the disc with obliteration of the cup).
   (c) *Arteries and veins*
      - Is there AV nipping of hypertensive retinopathy?
   (d) *Background*
      - Red lesions.
        Either haemorrhages or new vessels. (You should be able to distinguish between these at this stage.) Haemorrhages occur in both diabetic and hypertensive retinopathy.

- White lesions (exudates).
  Often described as soft (cotton wool appearance), as in diabetic or hypertensive retinopathy, or hard (small and intensely white), as in diabetic retinopathy and sometimes hypertension.
- Dark, pigmented lesions can be within normal limits if seen in isolated areas.
  Multiple patchy areas of pigmentation in retinitis pigmentosa.

(e) *Macula*

- Hard exudates in a star formation – macular star ★★ (hypertension).

Discussion points

1. Know the causes of papilloedema.
2. Know the causes of optic atrophy.
3. Explain why the macula is important.

BLACKOUTS ★★★★

No strict definition for blackouts can be made; indeed, patients will have very different ideas of what a blackout is. Nevertheless, a proposed differentiation of syncope from falls is listed. Bear in mind that around 30% of older adults with true syncope may present with unexplained falls and deny loss of consciousness. Blackouts are a very common presenting disorder, and your ability to obtain a good history will be crucial.

DEFINITIONS

- **Syncope** Transient loss of consciousness with loss of postural tone.

- **A fall** Coming to rest on the ground with no loss of consciousness.
- **Epilepsy** A condition in which there is intermittent abnormal electrical activity within the brain.

CAUSES OF BLACKOUTS

Neurological ★★★
- Epilepsy   ★★★★
- Vertebrobasilar ischaemia   ★★★
- Ménière's disease   ★

Cardiac ★★★★
- Painless MI   ★★★
- Vasovagal syncope   ★★★
- Aortic stenosis   ★★★
- Arrhythmias   ★★★
- Postural hypotension   ★★★
- Stokes–Adams attacks   ★★★

Miscellaneous ★
- Drugs
    - Insulin/oral hypoglycaemics   ★
    - antihypertensives   ★★★
    - glyceryl trinitrate   ★★
    - tricyclics   ★
    - L-dopa   ★
- Hyperventilation
- Drop attacks
- GI haemorrhage
- Alcohol

HISTORY

Try to decide whether the blackout is secondary to cardiac or neurological disease. Establish what the patient means by a 'blackout' and the circumstances in which they occur (e.g. after coughing or micturition). How frequent are they and how long do they last? How does the patient feel afterwards (e.g. postictal/injuries)? Does the patient lose consciousness? Is the patient pale or cyanosed? Have eye-witnesses told the patient what they have seen (up to 50% will have no eye-witness account)? Is there a warning to the attack? Are there other features? Have injuries been sustained? Syncope during exertion suggests aortic outflow obstruction or ischaemic heart disease. Vertigo suggests vertebrobasilar ischaemia. Symptoms on standing suggest postural hypotension. Also, enquire about significant past medical history and drug history. A history of cardiac disease strongly points to a CVS cause of blackout.

EXAMINATION

Examination may be unhelpful, but cardiac and neurological examinations may reveal the cause. Listen for carotid bruit and check lying and standing BPs. Listen for murmurs or evidence of heart failure. Is there any evidence of cerebral ischaemia?

FACTFILE

1. Syncope is common but its causes are difficult to diagnose. In approximately 20–30% of cases the underlying cause remains unknown and, especially in the elderly, there may be more than one contributing factor. Syncope is not benign: the 1-year mortality for cardiovascular syncope is 20%!

2. Investigations: ECG and echo will establish whether there is structural heart disease (and by implication suggest a cardiac cause of syncope); 24-hour ECG should be performed but this is often unhelpful if syncope occurs infrequently. Exercise

tolerance testing should be considered if syncope or presyncope occurs on exertion.

3. EEG and CT brain should be considered if seizures or cerebrovascular ischaemia is likely.

4. Painless MI may occur in up to 20% of cases. This is usually in the elderly, diabetics and hypertensives.

5. Once symptoms arise from aortic stenosis, the prognosis is poor; investigation with a view to valve replacement should therefore be considered.

6. Epilepsy has a prevalence of 0.5–1% of the population. It is more common in childhood and older age.

7. Most doctors would not consider treatment with anticonvulsants after a single seizure. Some patients with very infrequent seizures may not wish to take anticonvulsants.

8. In patients with uncontrolled epilepsy, remember non-compliance with anticonvulsants as a possible cause. An incorrect diagnosis should also be considered.

9. A diagnosis of epilepsy has major life-style implications (e.g. work, driving, recreation).

Discussion points

1. Be prepared to discuss investigation of syncope. This should be influenced by the most likely cause on the basis of history and examination. It would be reasonable to mention the need to question any witnesses as a possible further investigation – in many instances this will be the most fruitful 'investigation'.

2. Know the definition of status epilepticus (prolonged or recurrent seizures without regaining consciousness between fits) and how it is treated.

3. You may be asked to discuss the diagnosis of epilepsy with a 'first fitter'. This would test your communication skills, not only in explaining the condition but also in giving life-style advice.

4. What are the driving regulations for patients with a diagnosis of epilepsy?
5. Know the side-effects of the anticonvulsant drugs.

THE NEUROLOGICAL PATIENT (excluding blackouts) ★★★

The most likely neurological conditions you will encounter in the finals are discussed below. Be aware that these conditions are far more common in exams than in clinical practice:

- cerebrovascular disease (see p. 15)
- epilepsy   ★★★ (see p. 50)
- Parkinson's disease   ★★★
- multiple sclerosis   ★★★
- motor neurone disease   ★★★
- sensory neuropathy   ★★★

DEFINITIONS

- **Multiple sclerosis** A disease of unknown cause, characterized by multiple areas of demyelination in the brain and spinal cord. These are disseminated in both time and space.
- **Parkinson's disease** A progressive degenerative disorder of the extrapyramidal system, characterized by akinesia, rigidity and tremor.
- **Motor neurone disease** A disorder characterized by progressive degeneration of motor neurones in the spinal cord, cranial nerves and cortex.
- **Sensory neuropathy** A disorder of sensation due to disease in the sensory nerves.

HISTORY

Patients will often know the diagnosis and tell you themselves what is wrong. Ascertain whether symptoms have been gradually worsening or arisen acutely. Are symptoms symmetrical? Which functions have been particularly affected (e.g. optic neuritis in MS, swallowing in MND). How is the gait affected? Does the patient 'freeze'? Is there difficulty turning over in bed (as occurs in Parkinson's disease)? The presence of sensory symptoms excludes a diagnosis of MND. As always, find out what impact the disease has had on everyday life. Drug history may be relevant (parkinsonism, cerebellar dysfunction).

EXAMINATION

Important points may be observed during history taking (e.g. cerebellar speech in MS or the expressionless face of Parkinson's disease). Is there a pill-rolling or intention tremor? Full CNS examination should be performed but pay particular attention to those functions which the patient finds difficult. Observe the patient walking. Is there a festinant gait, foot drop or cerebellar or spastic ataxia? If you suspect MND look for evidence of fasciculation (limbs and tongue) and bulbar dysfunction. If you are asked to test sensory function give clear instructions to the patient and check pinprick, light touch, vibration and proprioception.

FACTFILE

1. Multiple (disseminated) sclerosis cannot be diagnosed after a single isolated symptom. The lesions must be disseminated in both time and place.

2. As with many diseases, MS usually follows a relapsing and remitting course but approximately 15% of patients have chronically progressive disease without remission.

3. MRI scans can now detect areas of demyelination but these are not diagnostic in themselves. CSF electrophoresis reveals

oligoclonal bands. In patients with previous optic neuritis, visual evoked responses may be prolonged.

4. Urinary symptoms, including incontinence, are common in MS. In patients with an acute deterioration, urinary tract infection should be excluded.

5. MS has no cure but there is some evidence that short courses of steroids can reduce the length of relapses but do not modify progression of disease. The role of interferon beta is controversial and it is expensive.

6. Spasticity can be painful and is usually treated with baclofen and/or benzodiazepines.

7. Physiotherapy should be offered to all patients with MS.

8. Parkinsonism, of which PD is one cause, is a syndrome of tremor, rigidity and bradykinesia.

9. Neuroleptics are the commonest drug-induced cause of parkinsonism.

10. Treatment of PD should be with the lowest possible dose of drug to avoid side-effects.

11. Depression and dementia commonly occur in PD.

12. MND has no known cause or treatment. Survival for more than 3 years is almost unheard of. The focus of attention should be to assist with ADL.

13. Fasciculation is caused by spontaneous contractions of large muscle groups and is suggestive of lower motor neurone disorders.

14. Sensory neuropathy usually occurs in a 'glove and stocking' distribution, with the lower limbs more frequently affected. Reflexes will be diminished or absent.

15. Most common causes of a sensory neuropathy are diabetes and alcohol. Other causes include vitamin B deficiencies and certain drugs.

Discussion points

1. How does MS commonly present, what are the favourable prognostic features and what benefits do corticosteroids confer?
2. Be prepared to discuss which agents can be used to treat PD and the side-effects of L-dopa therapy.
3. Which drugs can cause parkinsonism?
4. Know the three patterns of MND: progressive muscular atrophy (~25%), amyotrophic lateral sclerosis (~50%) and bulbar palsy (~25%).
5. Be sure to know your dermatomes!

CRANIAL NERVES ★★★

Cranial nerve examination lends itself to inclusion in an OSCE. For brevity, and because certain cranial nerve lesions are rare, you are unlikely to be asked to examine the cranial nerves in their entirety. If you are very unlucky, you may be examined by a neurologist. On the other hand, you may be very lucky and be examined by a cardiologist whose skill in cranial nerve examination is rather limited. Obviously you are more likely to impress the latter if you look even vaguely competent!

HISTORY

You are likely to be given a single-sentence history and instruction to proceed with examination.

EXAMINATION

The abnormality may be obvious on general inspection. You must be prepared to undertake full examination of all the cranial nerves.

FACTFILE

1. The commonest causes of isolated cranial nerve lesions are: diabetes, MS, sarcoid, tumour and trauma.

2. In optic nerve lesions (e.g. optic neuritis) the direct light reflex is lost (sensory arc of the reflex is interrupted) but the consensual light reflex is preserved.

3. Holmes–Adie syndrome is a benign common condition in which the light reflexes appear absent and accommodation is sluggish and sustained.

4. IIIrd nerve palsy causes ptosis, and a dilated, non-reactive and 'down and out' pupil but bear in mind that the deficit may be incomplete and therefore ptosis may be absent.

5. IIIrd nerve palsy is an ominous sign if there is raised intracranial pressure.

6. IVth nerve lesions cause superior oblique muscle paralysis. This results in diplopia on looking down (walking downstairs is difficult).

7. VIth nerve lesions cause paralysis of the lateral rectus muscle and failure of lateral gaze.

8. VIIth nerve lesions can be subdivided into those of the upper and lower motor neurone. UMN lesions (stroke) spare the forehead due to bilateral cortical representation. If an LMN lesion is present, all of one half of the face will be affected. The most common cause in an exam will be Bell's palsy but look for the scars of parotid or mastoid surgery.

9. Bell's sign (LMN VIIth palsy): the ipsilateral eye deviates upwards on asking the patient to close that eye.

10. Rinne's test. Hold a vibrating tuning fork on the mastoid process until it is no longer heard. Then hold it at the external auditory meatus and it will be heard, i.e. air conduction is better than bone conduction (normal or sensorineuronal deafness). If bone conduction is better than air conduction this suggests a conduction deficit (e.g. wax, otosclerosis).

11. Weber's test. Place a vibrating tuning fork in the middle of the forehead. It should be heard equally in each ear. In conduction deafness it will be heard better in the deaf ear. In sensorineural deafness (trauma, VIIIth nerve lesion, infection) it will not be heard in the affected ear.

12. Bulbar palsy is caused by bilateral LMN lesions of cranial nerves IX, X and XII. It is most often seen in MND, when patients complain of regurgitation. Tongue fasciculation should be expected.

13. Pseudobulbar palsy is caused by bilateral UMN lesions (CVA). Patients have characteristic (Donald Duck) speech and may be emotionally labile.

14. Horner's syndrome consists of pupillary constriction, enopthalmos, ptosis and anhydrosis (loss of sweating). It is caused by interruption of the sympathetic nerve supply of the face. Causes include Pancoast (bronchial) tumour, syringomyelia, syringobulbia, sympathectomy and neck tumours.

Discussion points

1. Know the optic pathway (practice drawing this) and be able to explain visual field defects.
2. Know the subdivisions of the trigeminal nerve.
3. Be familiar with the external ocular muscles and how gaze is coordinated.
4. Be able to offer some causes of optic atrophy.
5. What are the features of raised intracranial pressure?
6. Explain how you differentiate an LMN facial lesion from UMN pathology.

THE PATIENT WITH WEIGHT LOSS / DEBILITY ★★★

Patients under investigation for these symptoms are ideal long cases, requiring the candidate to draw out the most likely cause(s) from an extensive list of possibilities. The history can be targeted provided you are aware of the potential causes. If there is an obvious clinical finding, such as hepatomegaly or a goitre, you may encounter such patients at an OSCE station. Many of these conditions will be covered individually.

CAUSES

With anorexia
- Occult malignancy ★★★★★
- Infective endocarditis ★★★
- Severe congestive cardiac failure ★★★★
- Alcoholism ★★★
- Tuberculosis ★★★★
- Uraemia ★★★
- Rheumatoid disease ★★★
- Malabsorption/inflammatory bowel disease
- Psychiatric causes (depression, dementia, anorexia nervosa) ★
- Neurological disease (e.g. PD or MND) ★★

Without anorexia
- Hyperthyroidism ★★★
- Diabetes mellitus ★★★★

HISTORY

Remember that approximately 80% of diagnoses will be made from the history. First, establish whether the patient has lost his or her appetite. This will direct you to the above list(s). Important points in the history would be the presence of altered bowel habit, dysphagia, cough, haemoptysis or

MEDICINE

dyspnoea. A history of cigarette and alcohol consumption is important. A past medical history of rheumatic fever or ischaemic heart disease should be noted. Also, try to obtain an estimate of the severity of weight loss and over what time period it has occurred. Many patients will be uncertain of how much weight has been lost but will be able to tell you if clothes are looser fitting.

EXAMINATION

Areas worthy of special attention may be evident from the history. Look for objective evidence of weight loss. Pigmentation (jaundice, uraemia) or lack of it (anaemia), clubbing and lymphadenopathy should be noted. Is there a thyroid mass? Thereafter, each system should be examined in turn. During examination the CVS should be assessed for new murmurs or evidence of CCF. Respiratory examination may reveal evidence of neoplasia or persistent infection. Abdominal examination may be fruitful, revealing hepatosplenomegaly (haematological malignancy), ascites or right iliac fossa mass (caecal carcinoma/Crohn's disease). Do not perform a rectal examination but make sure you tell the examiners that you would wish to.

FACTFILE

1. A massively enlarged spleen will almost certainly be due to chronic myeloid leukaemia or myelofibrosis. Kala-azar and malaria are uncommon in the UK so don't offer either as your first cause of splenomegaly.

2. Virchow's node is found in the left supraclavicular fossa and is associated with gastric carcinoma.

3. If you detect lymphadenopathy be sure to describe not only the location of the nodes but the size, shape consistency, tenderness and inflammation. Tenderness and inflammation are

suggestive of infection. Hard nodes with skin tethering are more likely to be malignant. Lymphoma nodes are described as rubbery.

4. Tuberculosis is on the increase again. Drug resistance is now becoming a problem. TB is more common in the homeless, immunosuppressed, alcoholics and immigrants from the Indian subcontinent.

5. In a patient with general malaise and a predisposing cardiac abnormality, the possibility of infective endocarditis should be thoroughly pursued. The most common source of infection in endocarditis is poor oral hygiene.

6. Patients will usually 'underestimate' their alcohol consumption. In general you can multiply by 2 for a more accurate assessment of a patient's consumption.

Discussion points

1. Be prepared to discuss the investigation of patients with unexplained weight loss and debility. Try to be logical and don't offer the 'smokescreen' list of all possible investigations. Remember, a lot of information can be gained from the simple tests, e.g. FBC, CXR, ESR, LFTs and blood cultures. CT and MRI scans are never your first investigation of choice. Investigation strategy should be determined by physical findings or symptoms localized to a particular system or organ (e.g. if a history of altered bowel habit is elicited, discuss the need for rectal/colonic assessment).

2. Why might the incidence of TB be on the increase and why might drug resistance occur?

3. How would you confirm a suspected case of infective endocarditis?

4. In a patient with infective endocarditis, what are the possible sources of infection?

MEDICINE

SKIN DISEASE ★★★

Dermatology patients are often included in final exams for two reasons: they usually are otherwise well, give a good history and have obvious signs; they are often bored in the dermatology ward and will volunteer for almost anything in an effort to change scenery for a few hours.

The conditions most likely to be encountered in the finals are:

- psoriasis ★★★
- dermatitis/eczema ★★★
- drug-induced reaction ★★★
- neurofibromatosis ★★★
- vasculitis ★★
- occasionally, malignant melanoma ★★

HISTORY

Determine the time course and extent of the disease (including scalp involvement) and what agents have been in contact with the skin, e.g. domestic, industrial or therapeutic. Are there other symptoms such as pain or itch? It is also important to establish the impact of the condition on day-to-day life (for example, application of coal tar). Never forget to take a full drug history. Think of possible underlying disease which may be associated, e.g. eczema and asthma. Precipitating factors such as heat or sunlight should be sought. A family history may be of relevance.

EXAMINATION

As with any clinical examination, valuable information can be obtained from the end of the bed. We are often told to use our eyes, but if you have to examine a patient with a dermatological condition, then you should also use your sense of smell – if the patient smells of coal tar then the diagnosis is usually psoriasis. Make sure to examine all areas, including the scalp, mucous membranes and nails. Look for evidence of excoriation. Be able to describe the distribution and pattern of the disease, e.g. linear, ring lesions (see table). Specific terms used in the description of lesions should be used, e.g. macule, papule, vesicle, etc. Note that psoriasis usually affects extensor surfaces, whereas eczema predominates in flexor aspects. If the diagnosis is psoriasis, look for nail and arthritic changes. The presence of a vasculitic rash should direct you to the possibility of connective tissue diseases.

Descriptive terms in dermatology	
Macule	Flat, non-palpable, circumscribed lesion
Papule	Small (<0.5 cm) palpable, circumscribed lesion
Nodule	Large papule (>0.5 cm)
Excoriation	Scratch mark
Bulla	Large fluid-filled blister
Vesicle	Small fluid-filled blister
Petechia	Small macule of blood
Purpura	Larger papule or macule of blood; does not blanch
Plaque	Large flat-topped palpable lesion
Pustule	Pus-filled lesion
Weal	Itchy raised rash caused by dermal oedema

FACTFILE

1. Psoriasis affects approximately 2% of the population.
2. In psoriasis the skin proliferates at approximately ten times the normal rate.
3. Around 50% of patients develop nail changes: pitting, onycholysis, discoloration and subungual hyperkeratosis.
4. Psoriatic arthropathy occurs in approximately 7% of patients with psoriasis.

5. The presence of arthropathy does not correlate with the extent of skin involvement.

6. Lithium carbonate and beta blockers are recognized causes of exacerbations of psoriasis.

7. Eczema and dermatitis are interchangeable terms. Up to 40% of the population may experience eczema in their lifetime.

8. Eczema frequently presents with itchy erythematous scaly patches, particularly affecting flexural areas of the elbows, knees and neck.

9. Scratching can result in excoriation, skin thickening (lichenification) and secondary infection (if skin becomes broken).

10. Basal cell carcinoma (rodent ulcer) is the most common malignant skin tumour; it is locally aggressive but rarely metastasizes.

11. The prognosis in malignant melanoma is related to the depth of the lesion at diagnosis (Breslow thickness).

12. Neurofibromatosis is an autosomal dominant condition. Typically there will be café-au-lait spots, which are light brown macules >1–2 cm in diameter. There may also be subcutaneous nodules along the course of peripheral nerves.

Discussion points

1. A multitude of drugs can cause skin reactions – be aware of the most common associations. Please note, however, that answering 'Antibiotics' will immediately be followed by 'Which ones?'

2. Be prepared to discuss alternatives to coal tar in the treatment of psoriasis.

3. Ensure you can have an informed discussion about allergens that cause dermatitis and the management options.

4. Be in a position to offer some of the associations of neurofibromatosis.

DIARRHOEA ★★★

Diarrhoea can be defined as an increase in stool weight and/or frequency, but individual patients may interpret this symptom differently. You are unlikely to meet a case of diarrhoea as anything other than a long case. The causes of diarrhoea are legion, but in the exam you are most likely to encounter:

- inflammatory bowel disease ★★★
- malabsorption ★★★
- infection ★★
- irritable bowel syndrome ★★
- colonic neoplasm (see p. 95)
- diverticular disease (see p. 95)

HISTORY

Identify what the patient means by diarrhoea. Determine bowel frequency, a description of the stool and whether blood is present. Steatorrhoea suggests malabsorption. Anorexia and weight loss suggest a possible neoplasm. Ask about tenesmus. An acute onset of symptoms points more to an infective cause or dietary indiscretion. If symptoms are chronic with a relapsing/remitting course, IBD should be considered. The major symptoms of Crohn's disease are diarrhoea, abdominal pain and weight loss. The major symptom in ulcerative colitis is diarrhoea with mucus and blood and only occasionally with abdominal pain. Systemic features of malaise, lethargy and anorexia are common in both ulcerative colitis and Crohn's disease. In severe flares, nocturnal diarrhoea, urgency and incontinence may occur. Manifestations of IBD other than gastrointestinal should be sought.

EXAMINATION

Look for evidence of weight loss and anaemia. Aphthous ulceration of the mouth is common in IBD. Abdominal examination may be unhelpful but a right iliac fossa mass and fistulae may be seen in Crohn's disease. Look for evidence of extra-gastrointestinal features, e.g. arthritis, iritis, etc. Although you should not perform a rectal examination, the examiners will expect you to acknowledge this as a crucial aspect of examination. Fortunately stool samples are not provided for inspection!

FACTFILE

1. Crohn's disease is a chronic inflammatory disorder which may affect any part of the GI tract from mouth to anus. Dentists not infrequently make the diagnosis (while examining the mouth!).

2. The following features suggest a severe attack of ulcerative colitis:
   - stool frequency >6 stools per day with blood.
   - fever (>37.5°C)
   - tachycardia
   - ESR >30 mm/h
   - anaemia – Hb <10 g/dl
   - albumin <30 g/l.

3. Even in patients with known IBD, never overlook the possibility of superimposed infection, especially if the patient is unresponsive to conventional therapy. Stool culture (including *Clostridium difficile*) should always be performed.

4. Some patients will require long-term oral steroids to control symptoms. In patients with proctitis it may be possible to administer steroids rectally to reduce the possibility of steroid side-effects.

5. Ulcerative colitis can be cured by surgery, whereas Crohn's disease cannot. Surgical intervention in Crohn's is indicated for symptom control.

6. Associations of ulcerative colitis include sacroiliitis, iritis, ankylosing spondylitis, hepatitis, cholangitis and colonic carcinoma (increased risk with extensive and chronic disease).

7. Coeliac disease is an allergy to gluten, a wheat protein. A life-long gluten-free diet is required.

Discussion points

1. Be prepared to discuss the differences (and similarities) between ulcerative colitis and Crohn's disease.
2. What are the complications of ulcerative colitis (or Crohn's disease)?
3. What are the side-effects of long-term systemic steroids?
4. When might surgery be indicated in IBD?
5. What are the histological features of coeliac disease and what foods contain gluten?
6. Know the major causes of infective diarrhoea.

DEMENTIA ★★★

Being asked to perform mental testing in a patient with dementia provides an ideal OSCE station or short case; however, you could be presented with a case of dementia as a long case in a psychiatry exam.

You should be able to discuss your findings and the potential causes of reversible dementia.

DEFINITION

A progressive generalized failure of higher cerebral function.

Incorrect answers to more than four of the following questions suggest a diagnosis of dementia:

1. Age?
2. Time (to nearest hour)?
3. Address for recall at end of test, e.g. 26 Smith Street?
4. Year?
5. Name of this place?
6. Recognition of two persons (doctor, nurse, etc.)?
7. Date of birth?
8. Year of the first world war?
9. Name of the Prime Minister?
10. Count backwards from 20 to 1?

FACTFILE

Assume that confusion / dementia is potentially treatable until proven otherwise. Divine Hatti may help in the exclusion process:

Degenerative (Alzheimer's disease)
Infective (CJD, syphilis, HIV)
Vascular / ischaemic (multi-infarct state, chronic subdural)
Iatrogenic (e.g. night sedation)
Neoplastic (cerebral tumour)
Endocrine (hypothyroid)

Hereditary (Huntingdon's chorea)
Autoimmune (hypothyroid)
Traumatic (recurrent head injury, boxers)
Toxins (alcohol)
Idiopathic (Parkinson's disease).

Discussion points

1. This will centre on the causes of dementia that are treatable. Know some of the above causes in case you are asked to discuss them in detail.
2. In practice, it is often difficult to tell whether a patient's confusion is new or of long standing when they are first admitted to hospital. Relatives may be helpful in clarifying this. Be aware of the causes of acute confusion in case you are asked to discuss these.

HEADACHE ★★★

This is unlikely to be presented as a long case. In an OSCE it is most likely to take the format of a case with an actor or patient.

HISTORY

A detailed history is essential in establishing the correct diagnosis. The commonest cause of headache is tension, but you should be aware of the salient features of other types of headache. Determine the exact location and character of the pain, associated features (e.g. photophobia or vomiting), precipitating factors (e.g. chocolate, cheese, shaving) and periodicity. Important points in the history are summarized below:

- sudden onset of occipital pain with neck stiffness – subarachnoid haemorrhage   ★★★
- unilateral throbbing pain, photophobia and preceding visual aura – migraine   ★★
- shooting 'electric shock' facial pain – trigeminal neuralgia   ★★
- temporal headache, age > 50 +/− visual upset – temporal arteritis   ★★★
- worse in the morning with vomiting and/or neurological signs – raised intracranial pressure   ★★★
- intermittent with nasal stuffiness and watery eyes – cluster headache   ★★
- headache with neck stiffness and pyrexia – meningitis   ★★★

Remember other possible sources of pathology such as sinuses, eyes, ears, temporomandibular arthritis and toothache.

MEDICINE

EXAMINATION

This is likely to be unhelpful as you will not encounter patients with meningitis, intracranial haemorrhage or acute migraine in an exam. Be prepared, however, to discuss important elements in the examination if you encountered the patient in a clinic or emergency department. This would include photophobia, neck stiffness, pupils and fundi. A full neurological examination should be performed.

FACTFILE

1. Migraine is the most common neurological complaint.
2. Remember the law of thirds in subarachnoid haemorrhage: one-third die, one-third rebleed and one-third survive.
3. A normal CT scan does not exclude a subarachnoid haemorrhage: examination of CSF is required.
4. SAH accounts for 10% of cerebrovascular disease.
5. Saccular 'berry' aneurysms account for ~70% of SAH.
6. Nimodipine, a calcium channel blocker, has been shown to reduce mortality in SAH.
7. Untreated, 25% of cases of temporal arteritis will result in visual loss due to inflammation of ciliary or central retinal arteries.

Discussion points

1. Be prepared to discuss poor prognostic features in SAH (e.g. age >65, coma, neurological deficit).
2. How would you confirm the diagnosis of SAH and how would you proceed with management?
3. Which individuals are prone to subdural haematoma?
4. What are the features of raised intracranial pressure?
5. Discuss the management of migraine, i.e. avoidance of triggers, prophylaxis and treatment of the acute attack.

THE ANAEMIC PATIENT ★★★

DEFINITION

Anaemia is present when there is a decrease in the Hb level below the reference range for the age and sex of the individual.

This may present as a long case, or as an OSCE station with a patient/actor or data interpretation of a blood film or FBC report.

HISTORY

Remember that anaemia is not a diagnosis (*cf.* heart failure) – a cause must be sought. Establish first whether there have been symptoms of anaemia or worsening of underlying disease, such as angina or intermittent claudication. Remember that the patient may have become gradually anaemic and therefore may be asymptomatic. Ask if he or she has been anaemic before and how it was treated. Pursue any history of blood loss (GI, menstrual) or altered bowel habit. A dietary history is essential. Is there any suggestion of malabsorption? Drug history should be noted (e.g. NSAIDs or cytotoxics). Past medical history will identify conditions associated with 'anaemia of chronic disease'. If the patient is not Caucasian think of haemoglobinopathies.

CAUSES OF ANAEMIA

1. Hypochromic, microcytic – Fe deficiency ★★★★★
2. Normochromic, normocytic – anaemia of chronic disease ★★★
3. Macrocytic – B_{12}/folate deficiency ★★★
4. Aplastic anaemia – congenital ★
   – acquired (idiopathic, drugs, radiation, infections) ★★★

5. Marrow invasion – e.g. lymphoma,
   leukaemia, secondary carcinoma ★★★
6. Haemolytic – Hereditary ★★ or acquired

EXAMINATION

Check conjunctivae and palmar creases. CVS examination may reveal tachycardia, hypotension (actively bleeding patients are unlikely to be exam subjects) or evidence of cardiac failure. Is the patient jaundiced (haemolysis)? Examine carefully for lymphadenopathy, hepatospleno-megaly and abdominal masses. Signs of chronic liver disease are noteworthy (?varices, pancytopenia). Inform the examiner that you would wish to perform a rectal examination and screen for FOB.

INVESTIGATIONS

The first line of investigation should be an FBC and film. Thereafter think of anaemia as microcytic, normocytic or macrocytic. Iron-deficiency anaemia indicates the need for GI investigation. If macrocytic, check vitamin B_{12} and folate (also TFTs). In older patients with a low B_{12}, a Schilling test is indicated. Investigation and treatment of normochromic, normocytic anaemia will be that of the underlying disorder. If haemolysis is present there will be an increased bilirubin and reticulocyte count, with decreased haptoglobins.

FACTFILE

1. Iron is present in meat, liver, eggs, milk and green vegetables.
2. Vitamin B_{12} is found in meat, fish, eggs and milk but not in plants.
3. Dietary folate is usually obtained from green vegetables.
4. Pernicious anaemia (PA) is associated with gastric atrophy and an increased risk of gastric carcinoma.

---

5. PA must be distinguished from other causes of B_{12} deficiency, e.g. vegan diet, terminal ileal disease or bacterial overgrowth in the small bowel.
6. Blood transfusion is rarely required in PA and may precipitate cardiac failure.
7. Pancytopenia (anaemia, leucopenia and thrombocytopenia) suggests marrow failure; examination of the marrow is required.

Discussion points

1. Be prepared to discuss how you would manage a patient with iron-deficiency anaemia.
2. What are the causes of upper GI blood loss?
3. Why are vegans prone to vitamin B_{12} deficiency?
4. Describe the principle of the Schilling test.

THE THYROID ★★★

In an OSCE you may be asked to assess the thyroid status of a patient from a brief history and examination or as data interpretation of TFTs. Alternatively, you may be instructed simply to 'examine the neck'. Rarely you may encounter a thyroid patient as a long case. Thyroid disorders are very common and increase with age. The diagnosis of thyroid dysfunction is biochemical but careful history and examination may point to the diagnosis. Remember, however, that only rarely will the classical picture of thyroid disease be present.

HISTORY

Any symptoms of hypo- or hyperthyroidism should be noted. Determine if there is a PMH of thyroid surgery or radioiodine treatment. Drug history is important (e.g. thyroxine, amiodarone, lithium, carbimazole). Ask about family history of thyroid and other autoimmune disorders.

MEDICINE

EXAMINATION

Examination of the thyroid gland itself is discussed in the surgical section of this book. On inspection look for evidence of a goitre, hair loss, tremor, exophthalmos or lid lag. Myxoedema may be present, i.e. subcutaneous mucopolysaccharide accumulation. Are the palms sweaty and is there a tachycardia or AF? Remember to listen for a thyroid bruit and check for retrosternal extension (inability to palpate the lower margin of the gland).

FACTFILE

1. Thyrotoxicosis can be treated with antithyroid drugs, radio-iodine and surgery. Radioiodine treatment is safe and appropriate in nearly all types of hyperthyroidism, especially in the elderly.
2. Radioiodine is contraindicated in children, pregnant patients and breast-feeding mothers.
3. The principal indications for surgery are pressure symptoms from a large goitre, the possibility of malignancy and for cosmetic reasons.
4. All patients treated with radioiodine or surgery should have yearly TFTs.
5. Carbimazole is the most widely used antithyroid drug but the FBC should be monitored as neutropenia can occur.
6. Thyroxine treatment should be initiated cautiously in patients with symptomatic IHD as the resulting increase in metabolic rate can precipitate unstable angina / acute MI.
7. Routine screening of the healthy adult population is not justified.

Discussion points

1. This will usually centre on symptoms and treatment of hypo- or hyperthyroidism.
2. What are the complications of thyroid surgery?
3. Be prepared to discuss other autoimmune conditions.

RENAL FAILURE ★★★

DEFINITION

A reduction in renal function with a consequent rise in blood urea and serum creatinine. Acute renal failure develops over days or a few weeks, whereas chronic renal failure develops over months or years.

You are unlikely to see a patient with acute renal failure as a long case. You may see someone with chronic renal failure attending for treatment. Alternatively, you may be asked to interpret a set of U&Es as an OSCE station.

CAUSES OF CHRONIC RENAL FAILURE

- Diabetes mellitus ★★★★★
- Glomerulonephritis ★★★
- Pyelonephritis / tubulointerstitial nephritis ★★★
- Hypertension ★★★
- Polycystic kidneys ★★★
- Drugs (e.g. ACE Inhibitors, NSAIDs, gentamicin) ★★★
- Calculi ★★
- Connective tissue diseases ★★
- Myeloma ★★

HISTORY

This should aim to determine whether the cause of renal failure is likely to be prerenal, renal or postrenal. Are there any factors predisposing to dehydration (e.g. diuretics, diarrhoea or vomiting)? Renal causes may be alluded to if there has been a previous history of renal problems or if there is systemic disease such as diabetes or systemic vasculitis. An accurate drug history is essential. Postrenal causes might be suggested by a history of prostatism or of cancer. Previous urinary calculi may be important, as may a history of abdominal or pelvic surgery. Always remember to document whether there are any symptoms of renal failure, such as nausea, anorexia, vomiting, fluid retention or hypertension. Ask if there has been dysuria, polyuria, haematuria or oliguria. If the patient is on dialysis find out the exact details and what impact this has on daily life. Finally, a family history is important.

EXAMINATION

As a long case make an initial assessment of hydration. Dehydration is suggested by reduced tissue turgor, low JVP and a dry-looking tongue. Check the blood pressure for postural drop or hypertension. Fluid overload is likely if there is oedema, a raised JVP or pulmonary oedema. General inspection will reveal pallor or the characteristic lemon-yellow tinge. A vasculitic rash or evidence of pruritus may be apparent. Abdominal examination should document whether there is loin tenderness (tubulonephritis) or renal enlargement (polycystic kidneys) or palpable bladder (prostate or pelvic pathology). Inform the examiners of the necessity of performing a rectal examination. Never forget to perform urinalysis if a sample is present. Note the presence of an AV fistula. This may in fact be a clinical sign as an OSCE station.

FACTFILE

1. Dialysis should be considered when K^+ >6 mmol/l, urea >40, fluid overload, HCO <12 and creatinine >500 μmol/l.
2. Continuous ambulatory peritoneal dialysis is easy to teach, less expensive than haemodialysis in the short term, can be performed easily with less social inconvenience (e.g. holidays) and is less time-consuming. Disadvantages include peritonism

(50% in 2 years need to discontinue CAPD), weight gain, hernias and pancreatitis.

3. Haemodialysis is more time-consuming, requiring time off work, etc.

4. Haemorrhage, hepatitis, sepsis and cerebral oedema are recognized complications of haemodialysis.

5. Roughly 50% of haemodialysis patients in the UK have home haemodialysis; this alleviates some of these problems but obviously has cost implications.

6. Most patients require 12–21 hours of dialysis per week in 2–3 sessions.

7. Human recombinant erythropoietin is useful in the treatment of anaemia in chronic renal failure. Side-effects include hypertension, clotting problems and convulsions.

Discussion points

1. Know how to perform a 24-hour urine sample. 'Instruct this patient in how to perform a 24-hour urine collection' would be a good starting point in a communication station.

2. Be prepared to discuss the clinical assessment of a patient's fluid balance and know about CVP monitoring.

3. Know the common causes of renal failure requiring dialysis.

4. What are the advantages and disadvantages of haemodialysis and peritoneal dialysis?

5. What are the problems associated with renal transplantation?

6. Other than fluid balance, what regulatory functions does the kidney perform?

DATA INTERPRETATION

As mentioned throughout this text, you are likely to encounter an OSCE station where you are asked to interpret data. In general medicine this will probably be in the form of blood tests, an X-ray (probably a CXR) or an ECG. Typical examples and tips to the aetiology are given below.

BLOOD TESTS

FBC

1. *Anaemia* ★★★★★
   - Low MCV (iron-deficiency anaemia / thalassaemia)
   - Normal MCV (anaemia of chronic disease – ESR may be of interest)
   - High MCV (B_{12} / folate deficiency)
2. *Pancytopenia* ★★★ (i.e. anaemia, low WCC and low platelets)
   - Marrow infiltration, drugs
3. *Leucocytosis* ★★★ (raised WCC)
   - Infection, severe trauma, malignancy

Urea and electrolytes

1. *Dehydration*   Typically will have a raised urea with a normal / minor rise in creatinine. A similar pattern can be seen after a GI bleed.
2. *Renal failure and hyperkalaemia*   Be prepared to discuss emergency treatment of hyperkalaemia.
3. *Hypokalaemia*   Diuretics, prolonged diarrhoea or vomiting.

Liver function tests

1. Elevated GGT in isolation (alcohol).
2. Elevated GGT and alkaline phosphatase (gallstones / pancreatic Ca).
3. Elevated AST / ALT (hepatitis of many causes – remember Divine Hatti).

Arterial blood gases

If you are asked to comment on ABGs they are likely to show respiratory failure. Ascertain whether they were taken on room air or oxygen.

Type 1 respiratory failure

- Low PaO_2
- Low / Normal $PaCO_2$
- Caused by ventilation–perfusion mismatch

Type 2 respiratory failure

- Low PaO_2
- High $PaCO_2$
- Caused by ventilatory failure

Look also at the pH. A low pH signifies an acidosis: if the bicarbonate is low there is a metabolic acidosis (look for a fall in CO_2 as it is 'blown off' to compensate). If the CO_2 is high then there is a respiratory acidosis (i.e. type 2 respiratory failure), typically seen in COPD.

ECG

There are only a few ECG patterns you would be asked to recognize. These are discussed below. If you are unlucky you may be asked to record an ECG or describe how you would do this. Phoning the cardiac department and sweet-talking the technician is of course the correct method in real life but unfortunately examiners are likely to award few points for such a response.

Recording the ECG

The patient should be lying comfortably on a couch or bed. Tell the patient what you are about to do and prepare the skin by rubbing lightly. Apply leads to the four limbs. The chest leads should then be attached at the usual sites.

Atrial fibrillation ★★★★★

Discussion topics may include pharmacological treatment of AF, both rate and rhythm control.

Acute myocardial infarction ★★★★★

1. Look for the typical feature of ST elevation, which is the most likely abnormality to be encountered.
2. Site of infarct:
   - V1–V6 – anterior
   - V1–V3 – anteroseptal
   - V4–V6 – anterolateral
   - I, AVL – lateral
   - II, III, AVF – inferior.
3. Be prepared to discuss the management of acute MI.

Left ventricular hypertrophy ★★★★

1. Look for large voltage complexes. S wave in V1 plus R wave in V5–V6 >37 mm.
2. Causes: hypertension, aortic stenosis, hypertrophic cardiomyopathy.

Heart block ★★★★

1. Look for P waves which are not followed by a QRS complex.
2. Commonly seen after acute MI (especially inferior), which often resolves spontaneously. Most frequently due to conduction system fibrosis, which requires permanent pacemaker insertion.

CHEST X-RAY

Typical CXR appearances you may encounter include:

- pneumonia ★★★★★
- pneumothorax ★★★★★
- bronchial carcinoma ★★★★★
- pulmonary oedema ★★★★★
- pleural effusion ★★★★★

The 'normal' CXR

It is possible that you will be asked to comment on a CXR that initially seems normal. In this case you should consider the following conditions, which you may have overlooked at first glance:

- small pneumothorax
- straight left heart border (mitral stenosis)
- dextrocardia (check film is not reversed before diagnosing this)
- mastectomy
- skeletal deformity (e.g. rib fractures or bony metastases)
- air under diaphragm
- genuine normal CXR.

SURGERY

HISTORY AND EXAMINATION IN SURGERY

This section is intended to be a guide to history taking in surgery. The majority of surgical cases in the finals will be of gastrointestinal problems. This section will focus on this. The list of topics is not intended to be comprehensive and in only a few patients will the history fit into an ideal mould. Where causes of certain symptoms are given, only the common 'top of the list' conditions are listed. You should refer to surgical textbooks for a full listing. It must also be remembered that, in common with the other specialties, surgical history taking encompasses the patient as a whole and, for example, medical disorders such as those already detailed will have an impact on surgical management.

THE CASES

DYSPHAGIA ★★★

DEFINITION

Difficulty in swallowing.

COMMON CAUSES

- Benign oesophageal stricture
- Oesophageal carcinoma
- Reflux oesophagitis
- Achalasia of the cardia

HISTORY

You may see this as a long case or as a standardized patient in an OSCE. You must establish the following;

1. Where does the food stick?
2. What type of foods are causing difficulty, i.e. solids alone or solids and fluids? If solids alone, is it certain types of food? Patients will usually have difficulty initially with dry materials such as bread. With total dysphagia, patients will have difficulty swallowing saliva.
3. Is the dysphagia progressive, and over what period of time? Rapidly progressive symptoms are suggestive of malignant pathology, whereas long-standing difficulty only with dry bulky foods would be more in keeping with benign disease.
4. Are there any other symptoms, e.g. weight loss, pain, respiratory disease, voice changes?
5. Is there a past history of reflux oesophagitis which predisposes to stricture formation?

EXAMINATION: LONG CASE

1. General: is there evidence of weight loss? Is the patient clinically anaemic?
2. Is there any palpable lymphadenopathy in the root of the neck or supraclavicular fossae?
3. Are there any abnormalities on abdominal palpation, in particular an epigastric mass or hepatomegaly?

INVESTIGATIONS

- Barium swallow
- Upper GI endoscopy
- Chest X-ray

UPPER ABDOMINAL PAIN ★★★★★

DEFINITION

Abdominal pain above the level of the umbilicus.

COMMON CAUSES

• Gallbladder disease	★★★★★
• Duodenal ulcer	★★★★
• Gastric ulcer (benign or malignant)	★★★
• Pancreatic disease	★★★

HISTORY AND EXAMINATION

As for pain in any other part of the body, you must determine the exact site, radiation, severity, character, associated features, precipitating and relieving factors. In many instances, once you have done this you should have a good idea as to the likely cause of the patient's symptoms. It is important to remember that rarely are any patient's symptoms 'typical' of a condition but the following may help to determine the underlying problem.

Gallbladder disease ★★★★★

Frequent complaints are of episodic upper abdominal pain, predominantly epigastric and right upper quadrant, which can radiate around to the back, the interscapular area, or to the right shoulder tip. With symptoms, the patient is restless and unable to obtain a comfortable position. Often he or she may complain that their symptoms are precipitated by eating and are accompanied by nausea and flatulence. Spontaneous resolution occurs after a variable period of time. These symptoms are frequently labelled as biliary 'colic', although they are more likely to reflect gallbladder distension rather than true colic. A separate clinical entity is acute cholecystitis, where there is mucosal inflammation and ulceration secondary to cystic duct obstruction. Local discomfort and tenderness is a feature of this condition, with systemic signs of toxaemia. On examination look for any evidence of jaundice. Check for tenderness or a palpable gallbladder in the right upper abdominal quadrant, often exacerbated by deep inspiration (Murphy's sign). Upper abdominal ultrasound is the first investigation of choice.

Duodenal ulcer disease ★★★★

The most common complaint of patients with chronic duodenal ulcer disease is epigastric pain precipitated by fasting and relieved by food or antacids. Not infrequently patients are woken from sleep by their symptoms. Sometimes the discomfort radiates through to the back, and certain foods (particularly strongly seasoned ones) or alcohol may aggravate matters. There may be a history of intermittent vomiting or previous haematemesis. Weight loss is uncommon in uncomplicated duodenal ulcer disease but symptoms of anaemia may develop from chronic upper GI blood loss. On examination, look for clinical signs of anaemia and check the abdomen for any palpable abnormality and tenderness. Investigation is by upper GI endoscopy.

Gastric pathology ★★★

Patients with gastric lesions frequently complain of a gnawing discomfort and vague dyspepsia. These symptoms are often constant and not affected by food or antacid mixtures. Profound anorexia is a common complaint, particularly in patients with malignant disease, and weight loss is a frequent feature. Intermittent vomiting and minor haematemesis are not uncommon. Proximal gastric cancers may result in dysphagia, whereas pyloric canal lesions can lead to gastric outlet obstruction. General examination should include a check for signs of anaemia, weight loss, and lymphadenopathy in the supraclavicular regions. When considering the abdomen you may need to determine whether a succussion splash is present, or whether there is any evidence of ascites. Palpate the abdomen and note if there is an upper abdominal mass, tenderness or palpable hepatomegaly. Initial investigations is by upper GI endoscopy +/– biopsy.

Pancreatic disease

See p. 91.

JAUNDICE ★★★★★

DEFINITION

A yellow discoloration of the skin and sclerae secondary to an elevated serum bilirubin.

Classification

- Prehepatic (or haemolytic)
- Hepatic
- Posthepatic (obstructive)

In a surgical ward or examination, the most likely type of jaundice is posthepatic or obstructive. It is essential, however, that you are aware of how to determine the probable type of jaundice clinically and what investigations to arrange.

HISTORY

1. History of presenting complaint and all other symptoms.
2. Is the urine dark immediately it has been passed (indicates the passage of conjugated bilirubin in obstructive jaundice)?
3. Are the stools pale (reflects the absence of bile pigments in obstructive jaundice)?
4. Is the skin itchy (occurs in obstructive jaundice due to the deposition of excess circulating bile salts)?
5. Is the patient known to have gallstones?
6. Is there a history of liver disease (e.g. viral hepatitis, primary biliary cirrhosis, etc.)?
7. Is there a history of any haemolytic condition (e.g. hereditary spherocytosis, thalassaemia, etc.)?
8. Has the patient previously had biliary tract surgery?
9. Has the patient had any other significant illness? A history of malignant disease might raise the possibility of liver metastases or nodal obstruction to the biliary tree in the porta hepatis.
10. Alcohol consumption. Is this excessive?
11. Drug history. Some agents are directly hepatotoxic (e.g. overdose of paracetamol); some can cause intrahepatic cholestasis (e.g. the oral contraceptive and phenothiazines); others can precipitate haemolysis.
12. Occupational history, particularly in relation to toxin exposure.

EXAMINATION

1. Establish that the patient is jaundiced, remembering that the earliest signs are in the sclerae.
2. Are there any excoriations suggesting itch?
3. Look for evidence of chronic liver disease.

4. Examine the abdomen, paying particular attention to the presence of ascites, hepatomegaly, a palpable gallbladder and any abnormal masses.

INVESTIGATIONS

Urine testing

Using standard multitest strips, this is easily performed in the ward and may form a station in an OSCE circuit. The presence of bilirubin indicates obstructive jaundice (or intrahepatic cholestasis), as only water-soluble conjugated bilirubin can pass through the glomerulus. Urobilinogen will be absent in total biliary obstruction because it comes from the gut following bacterial action on bile products. Excess urobilinogen will, however, be present in haemolytic jaundice.

Liver function tests

The bilirubin level will confirm jaundice and give an indication as to its severity. A disproportionately raised alkaline phosphatase is suggestive of biliary tract obstruction, whereas high levels of the transaminases (AST and ALT) are indicative of hepatocellular damage. As in Medicine, you may be presented with LFTs as a data interpretation station.

Coagulation screen

Coagulation will be normal in prehepatic jaundice. The prothrombin time will be often prolonged in obstructive jaundice but correctable with parenteral vitamin K (10 mg intravenously on three consecutive days is sufficient). In severe hepatocellular disease both the PT and APTT will be prolonged and the former will not be corrected by vitamin K.

Viral screen

This should be considered essential in all jaundiced patients.

Imaging techniques

Ultrasound is the initial investigation of choice and can image the liver parenchyma, the intrahepatic and extrahepatic biliary tree, the gallbladder and the pancreas. CT scanning or ERCP may be required in certain circumstances.

FACTFILE

1. *Causes of obstructive jaundice* You will almost certainly be asked about causes of obstructive jaundice and you should present them in their order of frequency. In the following list, the first two conditions are responsible for the majority of cases:
   - gallstones
   - carcinoma of the head of the pancreas
   - nodes in the porta hepatis
   - bile duct tumours (cholangiocarcinoma)
   - benign bile duct strictures
   - sclerosing cholangitis.

2. *Courvoisier's Law* 'If in the presence of jaundice the gallbladder is palpable, then the jaundice is unlikely to be due to a stone.' This rule relies on the premise that in gallstone disease the gallbladder wall is thickened and fibrotic and therefore unable to distend in the face of an obstructed biliary tree. A normal gallbladder, however, can become considerably distended when the distal obstruction is caused by a carcinoma in the head of the pancreas. The rule is, of course, not absolute, as clearly gallbladder disease and carcinoma can coexist.

ACUTE PANCREATITIS ★★★

DEFINITION

A condition characterized by autodigestion of the pancreas by its own activated enzymes.

It is unlikely that you will be faced with a case of acute pancreatitis but you may come across patients who have previously been admitted with an acute event.

CAUSES

- Gallstones
- Alcohol
- Viral (e.g. mumps, coxsackie)
- Trauma (including surgery)
- Drug-induced (steroids, thiazide diuretics)
- Hypercalcaemia
- Hypothermia
- Idiopathic

The first two causes are responsible for the vast majority of cases.

HISTORY

The patient will usually have presented as an acute surgical emergency following the sudden onset of severe constant upper abdominal pain that frequently radiates through to the back. Often patients find sitting with the knees drawn up to the chest the most comfortable position to adopt. Vomiting and retching are a common accompaniment. There may be a history of long-standing chronic alcohol excess or of 'binge' drinking. Alternatively, there may be a history of gallstone disease.

EXAMINATION

You will not be asked to examine a patient in the acute phase of pancreatitis but you may be taken to someone who was admitted with the condition several days previously.

On general examination, take note of the patient's general demeanour. Does he or she look comfortable or distressed? Is there any evidence of jaundice? Does the patient have a temperature? Is there any evidence of chronic liver disease?

Extravasation of blood in haemorrhagic pancreatitis may cause discoloration around the umbilicus (Cullen's sign) or in the flanks (Grey Turner's sign). On abdominal palpation, you would not be surprised to find some tenderness and guarding in the epigastrium but note also whether there is any palpable mass. The abdomen may be generally distended if an ileus persists; the absence of bowel sounds will confirm this.

FACTFILE

1. *Diagnosis* This is based on measurement of the serum amylase. A level greater than three times the upper limit of the laboratory's reference range is confirmatory.

2. *Assessment of severity* The amylase level gives no indication as to the severity of the disease. You should be familiar with Imrie's and/or Ranson's prognostic criteria, which assign patients either to a mild or severe group. The former almost invariably settle with conservative management. On the other hand, severe acute pancreatitis is a serious condition with appreciable morbidity and mortality rates.

3. *Investigations* All patients should undergo ultrasound examination of the pancreas and biliary tree to look for gallstone disease. In gallstone pancreatitis there is increasing evidence that early ERCP with sphincterotomy and clearance of the common bile duct can alter the course of the disease. Patients with severe acute pancreatitis will require a dynamic contrast-

---

enhanced CT scan to look for evidence of pancreatic necrosis +/– fine needle aspiration to determine if there is bacterial infection.

4. *Complications* These are almost confined to the severe prognostic group and include infected pancreatic necrosis, pancreatic abscess and pseudocyst formation. In the long term, patients may be rendered diabetic (pancreatic endocrine insufficiency) or may have to take oral pancreatic enzyme supplements to aid digestion and prevent steatorrhoea (pancreatic exocrine insufficiency).

ALTERED BOWEL HABIT ★★★★★

DEFINITION

A change in any aspect of defecation (frequency, stool consistency, etc.) compared with what is regarded as 'normal' by the patient.

This is a common symptom for inclusion as a long case in the finals.

CAUSES

- Colorectal cancer   ★★★★★
- Diverticular disease   ★★★★★
- Inflammatory bowel disease   ★★★★★
- Infection   ★
- Irritable bowel syndrome   ★★★

HISTORY

You must establish what is regarded as the patient's normal bowel habit, remembering that there is considerable individual variation in frequency of defecation. What is the time period over which the change has taken place? Has there been any possible precipitating cause (dietary change, travel abroad, new medication, etc.)? Are there any associated symptoms (rectal bleeding, excess mucus, abdominal pain, tenesmus, weight loss, etc.)? Is there a personal or family history of GI tract disease?

EXAMINATION

General

Is there any evidence of recent weight loss or clinical signs of anaemia, etc?

Abdominal

Is there any evident tenderness or abnormal palpable masses?

Rectal

Always mention this, although in the examination setting you will rarely, if ever, be asked to carry out a rectal examination. Specifically, you would be looking for any palpable abnormality or evidence of blood or mucus on the examining finger.

INVESTIGATIONS

Colonoscopy or double-contrast barium enema combined with flexible sigmoidoscopy are the fundamental investigations in the majority of cases. The choice between the two will be determined by a number of factors, including the availability and waiting time for both investigations and the endoscopic experience of the clinician. Some clinicians will tend to use barium enema/flexible sigmoidoscopy for new mechanical problems, such as altered bowel habit, and reserve colonoscopy primarily for investigation of bleeding and assessment/surveillance of inflammatory conditions. Colonoscopy may also be selected in preference to barium enema as the first-line investigation in young patients to minimize pelvic irradiation, particularly in female patients. It goes without saying, however, that abnormalities identified on barium enema require further investigation by endoscopy.

FACTFILE

1. In the middle-aged and elderly patient the diagnosis is colorectal cancer until proven otherwise, and almost all instances merit further investigation.
2. In the young patient non-malignant causes are more common but the possibility of carcinoma should not be discounted, particularly if there is a family history of the disease.

RECTAL BLEEDING ★★★★★

DEFINITION

The passage of blood per rectum.

This could present as a long case or as structured oral examination inviting you to outline how you might investigate such a case. A less likely scenario is to be presented with an actor working to a script. History taking is essentially the same as a long case.

CAUSES

• Colorectal cancer	★★★★★
• Haemorrhoids	★★★★★
• Benign polyps	★★★
• Diverticular disease	★★★★
• Inflammatory bowel disease	★★★★★
• Anal fissure	★★★
• Ischaemic colitis	★★

HISTORY

What is the nature of the bleeding (e.g. bright red, altered blood, clots, on toilet paper, in the pan or mixed with the stool)? Bright red blood suggests an anorectal source, whereas altered blood and the passage of clots indicates a more proximal cause. Does bleeding only occur with defecation or does it necessitate the wearing of an incontinence pad? What is the timescale of the bleeding? Are there any associated symptoms (e.g. altered bowel habit, weight loss, tenesmus, abdominal pain, etc.)?

INVESTIGATION

Clinical examination, and others as for altered bowel habit (see above).

DISCUSSION POINTS

1. Haemorrhoids are the most common cause of rectal bleeding but must not be assumed to be the source of blood loss without consideration of more sinister pathology, particularly in the middle-aged and elderly age groups.
2. Melaena (offensive black tarry stools) usually indicates an upper GI tract source of blood loss but can occur with caecal lesions.
3. Remember that GI bleeding can be sufficient to result in anaemia without being clinically obvious. Right-sided colonic pathology (caecal carcinoma, angiodysplasia) is a more common source of this type of blood loss than comparable conditions in the left colon. Such patients will prove FOB positive on testing.

ABDOMINAL EXAMINATION

Obviously some of the cases given earlier may appear within the context of abdominal examination but abdominal masses commonly appear in surgical examinations as clinical signs which can be found as short cases or as an OSCE clinical sign station. Specifically, this section will include examination of the liver, spleen and kidneys. Another favourite is the patient with ascites, with or without signs of chronic liver disease.

DEFINITIONS

- **Abdominal mass** Any abnormal mass palpable on abdominal palpation.
- **Hepatomegaly** Palpable enlargement of the liver.
- **Splenomegaly** Palpable enlargement of the spleen.
- **Hepatosplenomegaly** Enlargement of both the liver and spleen.
- **Ascites** Free fluid within the peritoneal cavity.
- **Succussion splash** A splash heard in the upper abdomen when shaking the patient.

EXAMINATION

As for any system, this should proceed in an orderly manner, i.e. inspection, palpation, auscultation.

Inspection

Initially you should aim to perform a general examination looking for signs relevant to GI tract disease. The examiners may intervene and ask you to confine your examination to the abdomen itself but at least you will have demonstrated logic in your thinking.

General examination

Look for signs of anaemia (pallor, poorly injected conjunctivae, etc.), jaundice (pay particular attention to the sclera) and weight loss. Consider the other systemic signs of chronic liver disease, for example gynaecomastia, testicular atrophy, loss of body hair and spider naevi. Pay particular attention to the hands and look for clubbing, nail changes, palmar erythema and Dupuytren's contracture.

The abdomen

1. Look for any previous scars and describe them accurately.
2. Ask the patient to cough. This has two functions: in the presence of a previous scar it may demonstrate an incisional hernia (or groin hernia); and a patient's reaction to a cough tells you whether there is any peritonism.
3. Watch to see if the abdomen is moving with respiration.
4. Is the abdomen symmetrical?
5. Are there any obvious masses? If so, does the mass move with respiration? An enlarged liver usually can be seen to do so.
6. Is there any abdominal distension? Fullness in the flanks tends to suggest ascites.
7. Are there any dilated veins on the abdominal wall? Veins radiating out from the umbilicus (caput medusa) are suggestive of portal hypertension, whereas dilated superior and inferior epigastric vessels may be indicative of inferior vena caval obstruction.
8. Is there any visible peristalsis or pulsation?

Palpation

You will immediately create a good impression with the examiners, irrespective of what findings you elicit, if you do the following:

- Position the patient correctly.
- Position yourself correctly.

- Ask the patient if there is pain at any site before laying a hand on him or her.
- Watch the patient's face throughout to witness the reaction.
- Proceed in an orderly manner.

The patient should be placed supine with only one pillow supporting the head. The entire abdomen should be exposed, including the groins, although it is customary to keep the genitalia covered. You must be on the patient's right and position yourself such that your elbow is at the level of the patient so that your forearm and hand approach the patient's abdomen horizontally. If there is no chair present you will have to kneel on the floor to achieve this position.

Begin with light palpation and proceed round all four abdominal quadrants in an orderly manner, watching the patient's face throughout. If he or she has indicated that one particular area is tender, leave that quadrant until last. During this part of the examination you are largely gaining the patient's confidence but you should note any guarding, tenderness or obvious masses.

All four quadrants are then deeply palpated, again with a flat hand but this time exerting more pressure. Sometimes it helps to place one hand over the other for this purpose. Both hands may be used to assess the size of any palpable structure. As before, ensure that you pay attention to the patient's reaction, particularly the facial expression, as this is often the best sign of local discomfort. Remember that it is 'normal' to be able to feel certain viscera, particularly in thin patients. Such structures include the sigmoid colon, the caecum, the aorta and the lower pole of the right kidney (*cf.* the left kidney which is impalpable unless diseased).

Deep palpation is followed by the examination of specific organs or for certain conditions as follows.

The liver

The anterior edge of the normal liver is occasionally palpable below the right costal margin. As the organ enlarges, it extends down towards the right iliac fossa; hence, when asked to palpate a patient's liver you should start here. The organ moves downwards with inspiration and use is made of this excursion during examination.

Palpation is carried out using the flat of the right hand placed across the right side of the abdomen at right angles to the costal margin. The upper edge of the hand is pressed deeply into the abdomen during expiration and maintained in that position while the patient inspires. A descending liver edge will be felt against the edge of the examining hand as the patient takes a deep breath in. If you are unable to feel the liver initially, then gradually work upwards towards the costal margin, each time moving the hand during expiration so that it is positioned deeply again before the patient inspires.

Record the size of the palpable liver in terms of centimetres below the costal margin in the midclavicular line and note the character of its surface, consistency and the presence or absence of tenderness.

Percussion can be used to confirm the position of the lower liver edge but is the only clinical method of determining the upper limit of the liver. Always percuss from resonant to dull in the midclavicular line, i.e. from below upwards in the abdomen and from above downwards in the chest. The upper border of the liver normally lies between the 4th and 5th intercostal spaces but may be pushed downwards by conditions such as emphysema.

The spleen

The normal spleen is impalpable. The organ has to be enlarged by a factor of 2–3 before it emerges from behind the left costal margin and extends downwards in the direction of the right iliac fossa. Like the liver, the spleen moves downwards on inspiration and the same hand movements are used to palpate it, starting from the right iliac fossa and working towards the left costal margin. An equivocal spleen may be made more obvious by rotating the patient on to the right side. The organ is characterized by its notched anterior border.

The kidneys

The left kidney is normally not palpable unless diseased but occasionally the lower pole of the right kidney can be felt, especially in thin females. The kidneys are best felt between two hands: one placed in the loin pressing anteriorly and one on the abdomen pressing posteriorly. A palpable kidney may also be felt to descend on inspiration.

You should remember how to determine whether a left upper quadrant mass is kidney or spleen as follows:

- You can get your hand above the kidney but not above the spleen.
- A band of resonance is evident on percussion over the kidney but not over the spleen. Resonance is caused by gas in the colon.
- The spleen has a notched anterior border.

Ascites

The presence of free fluid within the peritoneal cavity can be determined by the demonstration of either shifting dullness or a fluid thrill and you should be familiar with both techniques.

Shifting dullness relies on percussion and, as always, you must percuss from resonant to dull, i.e. from the midline towards the flank. In general terms it is advisable to percuss the left side of the abdomen, as the presence of an enlarged liver on the right side (which is possible in a patient with ascites) can mask the gas–fluid interface. The hand in contact with the abdominal wall should be parallel to the midline;

the point at which the percussion note changes from resonant to dull is marked with a pen. The patient is then asked to roll on to the opposite side (i.e. normally the right side), following which you should wait a few moments to allow time for the intraperitoneal fluid to redistribute itself. Percussion is then repeated and, if free fluid is present, the line of demarcation between resonant and dull will have moved.

To perform the test for a *fluid thrill* you need an assistant's hand, the ulnar border of which is placed lightly on the abdominal wall in the midline. The palmar surface of one of your hands is laid lightly on the lateral aspect of the abdomen while you 'flick' the abdominal wall on the opposite side with a finger of your other hand. If sufficient free fluid is present, the impulse generated by the sudden sharp contact of your finger is transmitted to the palpating hand as a fluid thrill.

The aorta

The aorta is normally palpable in the upper abdomen of thin subjects and there may be visible pulsation. An overlying mass may make aortic pulsation appear more prominent and you should be aware of how to distinguish this from a palpable aorta or visible aneurysm. The key to this is that the pulsation of the aorta (or of an aortic aneursym) is expansile (i.e. the pulse 'pushes' your hands apart), whereas transmitted aortic pulsation is not expansile. To estimate the diameter of the aorta or an aneurysm, bring the radial borders of both hands together until you clearly feel the expansile pulsation, then subtract 1–2 cm from the distance between them to allow for the thickness of the patient's abdominal wall fat. Remember that the aorta bifurcates at approximately the level of the umbilicus and consequently can only be felt in the upper abdomen.

Auscultation

One of the few times you may witness a surgeon using a stethoscope is when listening for bowel sounds! All you really need to be able to do is to tell if they are normal (as will almost always be the case in an examination), absent (e.g. paralytic ileus or generalized peritonitis) or increased (intestinal obstruction). In the late stages of obstruction, when the bowel loops are distended, fluid-filled and atonic, there may be tinkling sounds caused by the movement of fluid from one distended loop to another. Remember that normal bowel sounds may be increased by a meal or by fasting.

Bruits caused by turbulent flow in a diseased aorta may be heard in the epigastrium. Be careful, however, that you are not simply hearing transmitted sound from a cardiac murmur. Disease in the iliac vessels may produce bruits along a line from the umbilicus to the midinguinal point.

The presence of a succussion splash in a fasted patient is diagnostic of gastric outlet obstruction. It is caused by excess fluid in a dilated stomach moving from side to side when you shake the patient. When present, it can usually be heard without a stethoscope. A similar noise can be often elicited in a normal patient within a short time (1–2 hours) of a large meal or consumption of a large quantity of fluid.

NECK LUMPS ★★★★

Neck lumps commonly appear in undergraduate examinations and are frequently a cause of great concern to candidates. Textbooks tend to print rather daunting lists of differential diagnoses. This section is intended to simplify the approach to the examination and diagnosis of the more common types of lump to appear in surgical finals. Thyroid disease is considered separately.

DEFINITIONS

Neck lumps should be described with respect to their position as follows:

- **Midline**   The anterior midline of the neck.
- **Anterior triangle**   Anterior to the sternomastoid muscle.
- **Posterior triangle**   Posterior to sternomastoid.

Lumps must be also described with respect to all the criteria normally applied to any lesions, e.g. size, shape, character, mobility, tenderness, etc. In the neck, lumps superficial to the investing cervical fascia are no different from lumps elsewhere in the body and comprise sebaceous cysts, lipomas, neurofibromas, etc. More specific lesions, many of which are peculiar to the neck, lie deep to the cervical fascia and it is these that are discussed here.

MIDLINE NECK SWELLINGS

Midline lumps are solitary lumps that arise from unpaired midline structures. The two most common are thyroglossal cysts and midline dermoids.

Thyroglossal cyst ★★

This is the commonest midline neck swelling and usually presents as a painless, rounded cystic lump which moves on swallowing and protrusion of the tongue. It can occur anywhere along the thyroglossal tract, i.e. from the foramen caecum to the thyroid isthmus, but is uncommon above the hyoid bone. The cyst is freely mobile and the majority transilluminate. Occasionally they become infected and present as a thyroglossal fistula.

Midline dermoid ★★

This usually presents as a painless solid or cystic mass anywhere between the suprasternal notch and the submental region. The feature which distinguishes it from a thyroglossal cyst is that it does not move with protrusion of the tongue or with swallowing.

SWELLINGS IN THE ANTERIOR TRIANGLE

These occur in the space bounded anteriorly by the midline and posteriorly by the sternomastoid muscle. Lesions to be considered include the following.

Thyroid lumps ★★★★

These are described in detail on page 109.

Branchial cysts ★★

The majority of branchial cysts present in the upper part of the anterior triangle in young adults. The presenting features are variable. Most patients are aware of a continuous swelling but occasionally it can be intermittent. Pain occurs in approximately 30%.

The typical branchial cyst is soft and fluctuant to palpation and can be felt extending out from the anterior border of sternomastoid. Transillumination can rarely be elicited owing to the depth of the cyst in the neck. Treatment is by surgical excision; the cyst contains straw-coloured fluid with abundant cholesterol crystals.

Pharyngeal pouch ★

This is a pulsion diverticulum which emerges through the dehiscence of Killian between thyropharyngeus and cricopharyngeus on the posterior aspect of the pharynx. Usually the swelling appears on the left side of the neck but, if large, it may extend over the midline. Many patients are asymptomatic; others experience problems with regurgitation or dysphagia.

Salivary gland swellings ★★★

These can be due to inflammation (acute or chronic), tumour or duct obstruction with retention of secretions.

Inflammation

Mumps is the most common cause of acute parotid inflammation and usually causes bilateral parotid swelling. Acute parotitis in the absence of the mumps virus classically occurs in the debilitated postoperative patient but can occur in otherwise healthy individuals. In such instances it is probably the result of ascending infection related to poor oral hygiene.

Chronic inflammation is more common in the parotid gland than in the submandibular gland and is most commonly associated with duct dilatation and progressive acinar destruction (sialectasis). Attacks of acute discomfort and swelling shortly following eating are the result of the ducts being blocked by epithelial debris. Stone formation is unusual in the parotid but common in the submandibular gland.

Tumours

The pleomorphic adenoma or mixed cell tumour is the most common salivary gland tumour and the only one likely to appear in examinations. It occurs most frequently in the parotid gland and usually presents as an asymptomatic, firm, well-demarcated, unilateral parotid swelling. The lesion is treated by parotidectomy but it has a tendency to recur locally owing to the tumour branching out into the capsule in a lobulated manner.

Malignant tumours more frequently affect the submandibular and minor salivary glands than the parotid. Pain and, in the case of the parotid, facial nerve paralysis should alert one as to the possibility of malignancy.

Retention of secretions

The submandibular duct is more prone to calculi than the parotid duct. Obstruction presents as pain and glandular swelling precipitated by eating. Often the offending calculus can be felt in the submandibular duct on the floor of the mouth. Alternatively, it can be visualized by plain X-ray, as the majority are calcified and therefore radio-opaque.

As discussed above, when the parotid gland is affected by sialectasis, the duct may become obstructed by epithelial debris and cause similar symptoms.

Miscellaneous conditions
Sjögren's syndrome should be considered as a possible cause of diffuse bilateral parotid swelling.

Lymph nodes ★★★★★
Lymph nodes along the jugulodigastric chain may be enlarged secondary to inflammation or a neoplastic process and present as swellings in the anterior triangle of the neck. Remember to look for evidence of lymphadenopathy elsewhere and for potential local causes, e.g. lesions in the mouth, on the tongue or of the thyroid, etc. Consider also the possibility of TB.

Carotid body tumour ★
This is a rare but well-known tumour of the chemoreceptor apparatus at the carotid bifurcation. It presents as an oval painless lump along the carotid sheath at the level of the upper border of the thyroid cartilage. Usually they have a reasonable degree of lateral mobility but cannot readily be moved upwards or downwards.

Cervical rib ★
Palpable in the supraclavicular fossae, these fibrous or bony structures may be associated with neurological (somatic or autonomic) or vascular symptoms in the upper limb.

Miscellaneous
Rare causes of neck lumps include aneurysms of the carotid vessels, sternomastoid tumours and cystic hygroma.

SWELLINGS IN THE POSTERIOR TRIANGLE ★★★★

The most common swelling in the posterior triangle (simple skin lesions aside) is lymphadenopathy.

LONG CASE

Any of the above conditions could appear in a long case setting but the majority are more applicable to short case clinical examination. Malignant neck lymphadenopathy in association with symptoms of head and neck (hoarseness, for example), respiratory or breast pathology, etc., or dysphagia secondary to a pharyngeal pouch are, however, distinct long case possibilities. As is always the case, the obvious abnormality must not be addressed in isolation. A detailed systematic history and careful clinical examination are essential.

OSCE

Standardized patients could be included (real or actors) with symptoms similar to that described above for the long case setting. The most common format would, however, be as a practical station. 'This patient presents with a lump in the neck – please examine' followed by a series of structured questions. Any of the lesions above could be involved but the most common by far will be lymphadenopathy. Given the diverse nature of the pathology, neck lumps also lend themselves to the structured oral type of OSCE station in which preset questions will probe your knowledge and understanding of the pathology concerned. Finally, there is potential for a patient with a neck mass to be used in a communication station. For example: 'You are about to perform fine needle aspiration cytology on this patient's neck lymphadenopathy. I would like you to outline to this patient what is involved and seek the patient's consent.'

FACTFILE

1. The most common neck lump is lymphadenopathy.
2. Inflammatory or reactive nodes are normally tender.
3. An exception to (2) is TB; here the infection is chronic and tenderness of the nodes is uncommon.
4. Palpable reactive-feeling nodes in children can be regarded as normal.
5. Palpable lymph nodes in adults must be regarded as pathological.
6. In adults, the primary source of neoplastic neck lymphadenopathy is usually in the head and neck rather than in the chest. Full oral and otolaryngological examinations for such patients is therefore mandatory.
7. FNAC is the first-line investigation of choice for suspicious neck lymphadenopathy.

THE THYROID LUMP ★★★★

DEFINITION

A mass arising from the thyroid gland.

Typical patients

- Those with a solitary thyroid nodule
- Those with a multinodular goitre

Thyroid cases are ideal for examinations and can be used in all exam formats. Being relatively prevalent in the community, there is a high probability that you will come across such a case at some stage. A sound knowledge of the clinical features and relevant pathology of thyroid disease is therefore advisable.

LONG CASE

History

The following factors should be taken into account:

1. Awareness of swelling/mass? If so duration? Variance in size? Associated discomfort?
2. Any symptoms suggestive of hyperthyroidism or hypothyroidism?
3. Past history of thyroid problems?
4. Geographic factors, e.g. areas of endemic goitre where there is dietary iodine deficiency?
5. Any history of neck irradiation?
6. Any symptoms of tracheal (stridor) or oesophageal (dysphagia) obstruction or hoarseness suggesting recurrent laryngeal nerve involvement?

Examination
General
Look for evidence of thyroid overactivity (e.g. tremor, sweating, tachycardia, weight loss, nervousness) or underactivity (weight gain, puffy eyelids, pretibial myxoedema, etc.). Pay particular attention to the eyes in cases of suspected hyperthyroidism (lid lag, lid retraction, exophthalmos, etc.).

The neck
Inspect the neck from the front. Is there any obvious thyroid enlargement (goitre)? If so, is it diffuse or is there asymmetry between the two thyroid lobes? If there is doubt about the nature of solitary lump ask the patient to swallow (a glass of water will usually be present as a 'prompt'!). Is there any evidence of cervical lymphadenopathy? Palpate the thyroid gland, standing behind the seated patient. Ensure that the patient's neck is slightly flexed. Carefully palpate both lobes of the gland and the isthmus and determine whether you are dealing with a solitary nodule or a multinodular gland. Flexing the neck and rotating the head towards the side being palpated will relax the sternomastoid

muscle and facilitate palpation of the individual lobes. As during inspection, ask the patient to swallow while you palpate the gland. Finally, palpate the neck and supra-clavicular fossae for evidence of lymphadenopathy.

OSCE

Standardized patient
You could be presented with an actor who has a script reflecting symptoms of thyroid disease and you would be expected to ask the relevant questions as outlined for the long case.

Data recognition
Although more common in a medical rather than a surgical setting, you could be presented with a brief clinical history accompanied by data with respect to thyroid function, thyroid autoantibodies and investigative results.

Communications station
You may be asked to explain the need for surgery for a thyroid condition, obtain consent for the procedure, and outline the major postoperative complications to a 'standardized' patient.

Practical procedure
'This patient presents with an anterior neck lump; examine the patient and describe your findings', etc. Thyroid cases, particularly solitary nodules, are commonly used in traditional short case clinical examinations in a similar manner.

Structured oral examination
The investigation of thyroid disease and the pathology of thyroid tumours are topics that readily lend themselves to the structured oral type of OSCE station.

FACTFILE

1. Investigations
   (a) *Bloods* Thyroid function tests and thyroid autoanti-bodies.
   (b) *Ultrasound* Distinguishes solitary nodules from multi-nodular glands and determines whether a solitary nodule is solitary or cystic.
   (c) *Radioisotope studies* A thyroid scintiscan may help to determine whether a nodule is solitary or part of multi-nodular change. It also identifies whether a solitary nodule does or does not take up iodine, i.e. the 'hot' or 'cold' nodule, but this is of limited value in surgical practice. Radioiodine uptake studies are sometimes used to make a functional assessment of thyroid gland activity in cases of borderline hypothyroidism or hyperthyroidism.
   (d) *Needle aspiration (FNAC)* This may empty a cyst or be used to provide material for cytology. Interpretation of thyroid cytology samples does require considerable expertise, which can limit clinical application. It is im-portant to remember that cytology cannot distinguish a follicular carcinoma from a follicular adenoma.

2. Treatment
   (a) Most solitary nodules are benign and the majority are cysts or 'dominant' nodules within a multinodular gland. If a cystic lesion becomes impalpable following aspiration, the patient can simply be reassured and observed.
   (b) The risk of a solid solitary nodule being malignant is approximately 10%. Given the difficulties with the interpre-tation of FNAC specimens, conventional practice dictates surgical removal of the affected thyroid lobe in patients with solitary solid lesions (thyroid lobectomy).
   (c) The indications for surgery in patients with multinodular goitre or autoimmune thyroiditis (e.g. Hashimoto's disease) are diagnostic concern, pressure symptoms (e.g. stridor or

dysphagia) or cosmetic (large unsightly goitres). Otherwise these conditions are normally treated conservatively.

(d) Thyrotoxicosis can be treated by antithyroid drugs, surgery or radioiodine.

3. Risks of thyroid surgery

(a) *Nerve damage* The recurrent laryngeal nerves are intimately related to the lateral aspects of the thyroid gland and therefore are at risk during thyroid lobectomy. The external laryngeal nerve may be damaged while mobilizing the superior thyroid poles. This nerve innervates the cricothyroid muscle, paralysis of which affects the tension of the vocal cords and hence the timbre of the voice.

(b) *Hypoparathyroidism* Transient asymptomatic hypocalcaemia is common after thyroid surgery.

(c) *Bleeding* This is probably the best known complication of thyroid surgery. If bleeding occurs deep to the cervical fascia the expanding haematoma can obstruct the airway and cause progressive respiratory embarrassment.

MALIGNANT TUMOURS

Although this section concentrates on malignant lesions of the thyroid, a common topic for discussion, it should be remembered that by far the most common thyroid tumour is the benign follicular adenoma.

Tumours of the thyroid follicular epithelium
Papillary carcinoma

This is most frequently seen in young adults and carries a favourable prognosis with 5-year survival figures in excess of 90–95%. It usually presents as a solitary thyroid lump, although it is occasionally diagnosed following excision of a lymph node mass. The traditional surgical approach is total thyroidectomy combined with removal of any involved lymph nodes. Radioiodine scanning is then done and any uptake taken to represent occult metastases. In such instances therapeutic radioiodine is administered. As the tumour is TSH-dependent, surgical treatment is followed by suppressive thyroxine therapy (0.2 mg daily). Some surgeons advocate a less radical approach with total lobectomy only being carried out on the affected side, with subtotal lobectomy (or no surgery) for the contralateral lobe.

Follicular carcinoma

Most commonly encountered in the 30–50-year-old age group. Unlike papillary carcinoma, follicular lesions tend to spread by the bloodstream to the lungs and bone. The prognosis is poorer, with 5-year survival figures being in the region of 60%. Treatment is the same as the radical approach to papillary carcinoma.

Anaplastic carcinoma

This normally presents as a rapidly progressive neck swelling combined with voice changes, stridor and dysphagia. Treatment is symptomatic and may involve a combination of surgical debulking and radiotherapy.

Tumour of the parafollicular cells
Medullary carcinoma

This may occur sporadically or in association with multiple endocrine neoplasia (MEN) type II. Surgical treatment is by total thyroidectomy. The tumour is not TSH-dependent and therefore thyroxine is required in replacement doses only. Calcitonin levels are measured as part of follow-up.

Tumours of lymphoid tissue

Thyroid lymphoma is rare; when it does occur it is most commonly associated with Hashimoto's disease.

THE BREAST LUMP ★★★

EXAM INCLUSION

Patients with breast disease may be used in a variety of undergraduate examination formats. Outlined below are typical examples of long cases and various OSCE stations. The latter would be similar to short cases in traditional clinical examinations. You should be aware that a breast lump might be present as an incidental finding in a woman who is the subject of a long case examination for some other problem.

Typical patients

- Young woman (<30 years) with a fibroadenoma   ★★★★ (the 'breast mouse')
- Older patient (>50 years) with a palpable breast cancer   ★★★

Other less likely patients would be a 'perimenopausal' patient (45–55 years) with a palpable breast cyst and patients with locally advanced disease who may have other clinical signs (e.g. palpable lymphadenopathy, pleural effusion, etc.) in addition to the primary breast mass.

LONG CASE

This is most likely to be a patient with breast cancer. The emphasis will be on taking and presenting an accurate history and demonstration of your ability to examine the breast and axilla in a logical manner. Important factors in the history include when the patient became aware of the abnormality and any associated symptoms. It is also important to establish whether there any specific risk factors for the development of breast cancer. In this respect an accurate family history is essential.

History

1. Presentation: ?symptomatic, ?incidental finding while washing, ?found by partner, ?noted during health screening/well-woman examination.
2. Variation with menstrual or HRT cycle if relevant? If so, do breasts change with cycle?
3. Any nipple discharge? If so, is it blood-stained?
4. Past history of breast problems?
5. Family history of breast cancer?
6. Parity?
7. Age at first pregnancy?
8. Breast feeding history.
9. Age at menarche and menopause?
10. Oral contraceptive use, past or present?
11. Hormone replacement therapy?
12. Previous history of radiotherapy to the chest or multiple CXRs?
13. General health, etc.

Examination

Inspection

Ensure that the patient is undressed from the waist up and sitting up comfortably on an examination couch or bed. Look for any asymmetry between the two breasts, making allowances for normal slight variations in size. Are there any obvious lumps present? Are there any skin changes such as tethering (areas of dimpling), ulceration or oedema (responsible for the peau d'orange appearance in advanced breast cancer). Pay particular attention to the nipples. Are they at the same level and of the same appearance. If one or other is inverted, establish whether this is recent or long standing. Bilateral slit-like nipple inversion commonly occurs in association with the benign condition duct ectasia, whereas recent unilateral nipple indrawing may signify an underlying carcinoma. Is there evidence of nipple or areolar eczema which may indicate Paget's disease? Finally, is there any evidence of bruising suggestive of needle biopsy? If a core biopsy has been taken in addition to FNAC, a small incision will be present and the bruising is usually more marked. Then ask the patient to raise her arms above her head. This may make skin tethering or lumps more obvious. In addition, as a breast fixed by tumour to the chest wall will be less mobile, this manoeuvre may accentuate asymmetry. Any abnormality should be described with respect to its position in the breast. Imagine the breast as comprising four quadrants divided by vertical and horizontal lines through the nipple.

Palpation

This should be done with the patient lying supine and with the arms by the side. Ensure that you examine the patient in an orderly sequence, e.g. normal breast, affected breast, normal axilla, axilla of affected side, both supraclavicular fossae, both sides of the neck. Palpate the breast quadrant for quadrant initially with the flat of the hand. Begin with the 'normal' breast so that you get an impression of what is normal for the patient before moving to the affected side. If a lump is felt, it is palpated between forefinger and thumb and described with respect to site, size, shape, consistency, definition of margins and tenderness. Deep fixation (to pectoralis major) should also be assessed. To do this, ask the patient to place her hands on her hips and alternately press down and relax while you move the breast lesion at right angles to the direction of the pectoralis fibres (i.e. move the breast lesion from inferomedial to superolateral and vice versa).

Examination of the axilla

The right axilla is examined with the left hand and the left axilla with the right hand. The non-examining hand is used to support the weight of the patient's arm. Begin by gently palpating the medial wall of the axilla and then gradually advance the examining hand towards the apex. Both supra-clavicular fossae and both sides of the neck are then palpated for any evidence of lymphadenopathy.

OSCE

The most common format for this type of patient would be at a practical station, i.e. 'Examine this lady's breasts', in which case you would proceed as described under examination in the long case section. Less commonly you could be asked to take a history from a standardized patient (again as for the long case), or risk factors for breast cancer could appear in a structured oral setting.

FACTFILE

1. Symptomatic breast complaints are common but fewer than 10% of women presenting to breast clinics have breast cancer.

2. Breast cancer increases in incidence with age. The lifetime risk is approximately 1 in 12 and half of sufferers will die from the disease.

3. Malignant lumps tend to be ill-defined with irregular margins (as they are invasive), be firm, may be associated with skin changes (tethering, ulceration) and may be deeply fixed.

4. Benign lumps tend to be well-defined, may be tender and vary with the menstrual cycle (if present).

5. Breast pain is a common symptom but in most instances is not indicative of cancer. Pain is an uncommon feature with a malignant breast lesion.

6. Most breast cancers are ductal adenocarcinomas.

7. Triple assessment of breast lumps comprises clinical examination, imaging (mammography and/or ultrasound) and FNAC.

8. About 5% of women with breast cancer have an inherited predisposition to the disease. Recent advances in medical genetics have identified causative genes as *BRCA1* and *BRCA2*.

DISCUSSION POINTS (long case and structured oral OSCE)

1. **Treatment of early breast cancer**
   Think of this in terms of local treatment directed at the breast and axilla (surgery and radiotherapy) and adjuvant systemic treatment directed at all potential sites of disease dissemination (hormonal therapy and chemotherapy).

   (a) *Surgery (local treatment)* Removal of the primary tumour may be accomplished either by simple mastectomy or by wide local excision (lumpectomy). The decision between the two will be determined by a number of factors, the most important of which are the size of the lump in relation to the size of the breast, the position of the lump in the breast (centrally placed tumours require excision of the nipple and would therefore normally be treated by mastectomy) and patient (and surgeon) preference. It is standard practice to remove at least some of the axillary lymph nodes during breast cancer surgery. Many specialist breast surgeons perform an axillary clearance (i.e. remove all the nodes, usually below the level of the axillary vein). An alternative is to excise a representative sample of the axillary tissue, a procedure termed axillary sampling.

   (b) *Radiotherapy (local treatment)* It is standard practice following lumpectomy to administer radiotherapy to the remainder of the affected breast to reduce the risk of local tumour recurrence. Radiotherapy may be given after mastectomy if there has been invasion of the pectoralis muscle or if the primary tumour was very large or of high histological grade but is not required in the majority of cases. Axillary irradiation is avoided following full axillary clearance as this combination is associated with a high incidence of arm lymphoedema; however, radiotherapy to the axilla will be required if positive nodes are found in an axillary sample specimen.

(c) *Hormonal therapy (systemic treatment)* Tamoxifen (a competitive oestrogen antagonist) is of proven benefit in postmenopausal women in terms of reducing the risk of recurrence, prolonging survival and reducing the risk of a second cancer developing in the opposite breast. It is therefore standard practice to prescribe tamoxifen in a dose of 20mg/day to all postmenopausal women following surgery. Recent evidence has suggested benefit also in premenopausal women such that the drug is being increasingly prescribed to younger women. Finally, tamoxifen may be used as a primary treatment in elderly women who are unfit for surgery or who have inoperable disease.

(d) *Chemotherapy (systemic treatment)* Combination chemotherapy with CMF (**c**yclophosphamide, **m**ethotrexate, 5-**f**luorouracil) is of proven benefit in node-positive premenopausal women. Other indications and forms of chemotherapy are constantly being evaluated in clinical trials.

2. **Treatment of advanced breast cancer**

The aims here are to control symptoms and to prevent disease progression. Hormonal therapy is the mainstay of systemic treatment but on occasions chemotherapy may be required for symptomatic metastases. Radiotherapy is useful in the palliation of painful bony deposits. Surgery has a limited role in the treatment of advanced breast cancer but 'toilet' mastectomy may be required for control of the ulcerating breast mass.

EXTERNAL HERNIAE ★★★★★

DEFINITION

An external hernia is a protrusion of part of a viscus from the peritoneal cavity through a defect in the abdominal wall into an abnormal position.

TYPES OF HERNIA

The following types of external hernia commonly appear in examinations:

- inguinal   ★★★★★
- femoral   ★★★
- paraumbilical   ★★★★
- incisional   ★★★★
- epigastric   ★★★

EXAM INCLUSION

All of the above hernia types could appear at a practical station in an OSCE format or as a short case in traditional clinical examinations. Groin and incisional hernia patients could also be used as long cases or in other OSCE formats (standardized patient, communication station, structured oral examination).

In a long case setting, typical cases would either be a groin hernia (usually a male in the second half of life and often with coexistent medical problems) or a patient of either sex with an incisional hernia. Note that the term 'groin hernia' has been deliberately used here and will be applied to the history and examination of inguinal and femoral hernia throughout the remainder of this section.

In an OSCE, the most frequently encountered patients in undergraduate examinations are:

- males (any age) with inguinal herniae ★★★★★
- females (usually middle age to elderly) with femoral herniae ★★★
- patients of either sex (usually obese) with paraumbilical herniae ★★★★
- patients of either sex with incisional herniae ★★★★

Finally, remember that inguinal herniae are common in elderly men and so a patient acting as the subject of a long case examination for some unrelated clinical condition may well have a hernia present.

LONG CASE

Groin hernia ★★★★★

History

It is necessary here to establish an accurate history as to the nature of the presenting complaint itself (the hernia) and elicit a history of any coexistent medical problems which might have precipitated the appearance of the hernia, dictate the anaesthetic technique or affect the outcome of surgery. A good social and occupational history is also essential.

Points to be considered include the following:

1. Is the history suggestive of a hernia? Is the patient aware of a groin lump? Is the lump there all the time or does it only appear with coughing/physical exertion, etc.? Does the lump disappear on lying down or after overnight rest?
2. Symptoms related to the presence of the hernia (there may not be any!): local discomfort? any colicky pain suggestive of intermittent intestinal obstruction? is the hernia reducible?
3. Symptoms or conditions which may have precipitated the appearance of the hernia and which may compromise attempts at surgical repair: chronic cough? chronic constipation?
4. Symptoms of urethral obstruction, e.g. prostatism?

5. Excessive physical effort? Childbirth? Previous surgery? Wound infection?
6. The patient's general fitness for surgical repair: cardiovascular disease? respiratory disease? medication (including anticoagulation)?
7. Factors that impact on postoperative recovery and activity: social circumstances? occupation? etc.

Examination of the hernia

The following questions need to be answered during the course of examination.

- *Is there a hernia present?* Start the examination with the patient lying supine. There may be an obvious bulge present, particularly if the hernia is irreducible. If not, ask the patient to cough and look for the typical bulge of a reducible hernia as the intra-abdominal pressure suddenly increases. If you still cannot see anything convincing, ask the patient to stand and repeat the above manoeuvres. The diagnosis is confirmed by feeling a cough impulse. To do this, placed the fingers of the examining hand gently over the site of the hernia and ask the patient to cough.

- *If so, is it reducible* (most will be in examinations)? The question is answered simultaneously with the previous one. Remember that an irreducible hernia may not have a palpable impulse.

- *Is the hernia inguinal or femoral?* Whether you do this with the patient lying or standing is determined by the ease with which you were able to demonstrate the hernia. What you simply have to do here is determine whether the visible hernia and/or palpable impulse is above (inguinal) or below (femoral) the inguinal ligament. Remember that this structure runs from the anteriorsuperior iliac spine to the pubic tubercle. Correctly speaking, an inguinal hernia will emerge through the superficial inguinal ring, above and medial to the tubercle, while a femoral hernia will protrude through the femoral ring

123

which lies below and lateral to the tubercle. The tubercle itself, however, can be difficult to palpate in obese patients, although in the male you can usually feel the spermatic cord running over it.

- *If inguinal, is the hernia direct or indirect?* This is the classical examination question but is of little clinical value. Distinction between direct and indirect inguinal hernias on clinical grounds is notoriously unreliable. The exception to this is that if the hernia extends into the scrotum it is almost certainly indirect. The principle behind this part of the examination is to determine whether an inguinal hernia can be controlled by finger pressure over the deep inguinal ring (indirect) or whether the hernia emerges medial to this point (direct). To do this you must first reduce the hernial sac. One finger is then placed over the deep inguinal ring (1 cm above the midpoint of the inguinal ligament), the other hand is laid gently over the medial part of the inguinal canal and the patient is asked to cough.

Examination of the patient

- *General examination* As normal but with emphasis on factors that might prejudice surgical repair, make surgery more difficult or affect postoperative recovery, e.g. obesity.
- *Specific features* These would include features that might influence decisions regarding surgery or anaesthetic technique, e.g. cardiovascular and respiratory examination. If there is any suggestion of prostatic symptoms then you should say that a rectal examination is indicated (but would not be performed in an examination setting).

Incisional Hernia ★★★★
History

The history of the presenting complaint (the incisional hernia), coexistent medical problems, and social and occupational factors must be obtained in a similar manner to that described above for the groin hernia. Clearly the patient will have had previous surgery and an accurate history of this should be obtained in terms of the dates of operation, how many procedures have been carried out through the same incision, whether the procedures were elective or emergency, whether there were postoperative complications (wound infection in particular) and whether there have been any previous attempts at hernia repair.

Examination

Think of this as a possible diagnosis whenever you are asked to examine an abdomen on which there is a visible surgical scar. The hernia may not be obvious with the patient lying flat but will usually become apparent whenever you ask the patient to strain.

Take careful note of what scars are present and how recent they appear. Is there already an obvious swelling in relation to a scar? If so, gently palpate it and determine its size and whether it is reducible. If there is no obvious swelling, ask the patient to cough and/or raise the shoulders off the bed (without using the arms). Does a hernia appear? If so, now palpate the abdomen and define the edges of the defect. The size of the hernial orifice can be of major importance in determining the urgency of repair.

It goes without saying that examination should also elicit any other abnormality, as in all abdominal examinations.

The entire patient should be examined in a manner akin to the groin hernia patient.

Other herniae

Paraumbilical and epigastric herniae may occasionally be seen.

OSCE

External herniae are ideal for OSCEs and can be included in a variety of formats.

Standardized patient

You could be asked to take a history from an actor who has the script for a patient with a groin or incisional hernia. This should be undertaken in an identical manner to that described for the long case.

Communications station

You may be asked to obtain preoperative consent, for example, from a patient with a groin hernia. This would include focusing on the management of the hernia itself, taking into account the risk/benefit discussion of repairing the hernia electively versus the risk of emergency presentation were the hernia to be left.

Practical procedure

This is the most common station format for herniae in OSCEs. Any of the herniae discussed above could appear here, with an instruction such as 'This patient presents with a right groin lump. Please examine the patient and demonstrate your findings.'

Structured oral examination

Herniae could be included in this format. Examples would include discussion about the types of herniae, causes of incisional herniae, etc.

FACTFILE

Groin herniae

Approximately 75% of all herniae presenting to surgeons are inguinal, of which about two-thirds will be indirect.

1. *Treatment* The only effective form of treatment is surgical repair. Trusses are only applicable to elderly patients who are unfit for operation.

Hernia surgery has undergone change in recent years. There is a continuing trend towards day case surgery and in some instances this is performed under local anaesthetic.

2. *Emergency presentation* Patients with groin herniae may present as emergencies for a number of reasons:

   (a) The hernia has become irreducible. In these patients the hernia may be tense and a little tender but there are no abdominal symptoms or signs and there is no redness of the overlying skin.

   (b) The hernia has become obstructed. These patients will have the typical symptoms and signs of (usually small bowel) intestinal obstruction. The hernia will be irreducible and tender.

   (c) The hernia has become strangulated. Strangulation of bowel within a hernial sac is suggested when there is reddening of the overlying skin and marked local tenderness in combination with the symptoms and signs of intestinal obstruction. The distinction between simple obstruction and strangulation, however, can only be made definitively at operation. Emergency surgery is indicated for suspected strangulation.

3. *Differential diagnosis* The differential diagnosis of a groin hernia includes inguinal lymphadenopathy, saphenovarix, undescended or ectopic testis, hydrocele of the cord, lipoma of the cord and femoral artery aneurysm.

SCROTAL LUMPS ★★★★

DEFINITIONS

- **Hydrocele** ★★★★ A collection of fluid within the tunica vaginalis.
- **Epididymal cyst** ★★★★ Single or multilocular cyst lying within the epididymis.

- **Varicocele** ★★★★ An abnormal dilatation of the pampiniform plexus.

EXAM INCLUSION

Scrotal lumps are most likely to appear at practical stations within an OSCE or as short cases in a traditional examination format. At times they could be used in a long case setting but this is less likely.

EXAMINATION

When presented with a scrotal swelling, there are a number of questions you need to ask yourself as you proceed with the examination:

1. *Can I get above the swelling?* This is the critical part of the examination in terms of confirming whether you are dealing with a primary scrotal mass. If you cannot get above the swelling, then it is likely you are dealing with a large indirect inguinal hernia.
2. *Is the mass solid or cystic?* Solid masses include testicular tumours ★ and chronic epididymo-orchitis ★★★ (acute epididymo-orchitis is extremely tender and therefore unlikely to appear in an examination). Cystic masses are likely to be either hydroceles or epidymal cysts. Spermatoceles are less frequently encountered but are most common in the head of the epididymis. They tend to be softer than epididymal cysts.
3. *Can the testis be felt separately from the mass and, if so, what is the relationship of the testis to it?* With an epididymal cyst, a normal testis will be palpable anteriorly. In tense hydroceles it is often difficult to feel the testis but when it is palpable it will be posterior to the swelling. The testis will feel normal in the presence of a varicocele but will be irregular if the diagnosis is a testicular tumour.

4. *Does the mass transilluminate?* This is a characteristic feature of hydroceles but some large epididymal cysts also transilluminate. This technique may help to confirm the relationship of the testis to the mass.

5. *Is the abnormality altered by posture?* Varicoceles become visible and much more easily palpable as a 'worm-like' collection on standing. Remember that varicoceles are almost invariably left-sided.

FACTFILE

1. Hydroceles may either be primary ★★★★ (no obvious cause) or secondary ★ to an underlying testicular tumour or testicular/epididymal infection.

2. Testicular tumours are rare below the age of 20 and above the age of 40 years. Between these two ages, however, they are one of the most common malignancies and usually present as a painless testicular mass with or without an associated hydrocele. The majority fall into one of two categories:

    (a) *Seminoma* A homogeneous tumour, which occurs most commonly in the 30–40-year-old age group. It spreads via lymphatics accompanying the testicular vessels to para-aortic lymph nodes. Treatment comprises inguinal orchidectomy, radiotherapy to the para-aortic nodes (the tumour is radiosensitive), and in advanced cases chemotherapy with platinum-based regimens.

    (b) *Teratoma* The peak incidence of this tumour is in the 20–30-year-old age group and comprises tissue derived from all three germ layers. Teratoma has a tendency for haematogenous dissemination and not infrequently presents as symptomatic lung metastases. Treatment requires inguinal orchidectomy and chemotherapy. It is less radiosensitive than seminoma.

3. While a rare event, a rapidly progressive varicocele in adult life can be secondary to renal carcinoma with thrombosis of the left renal vein or inferior vena cava.

VARICOSE VEINS ★★★★★

DEFINITION

Varicose veins are dilated, tortuous, lengthened superficial veins.

EXAM INCLUSION

The typical inclusion of varicose veins is as a traditional short case examination or as a practical station in an OSCE. A patient with varicose veins could, however, appear as a long case, particularly if there were complications (e.g. skin changes) or predisposing factors. Varicose veins could also be an incidental finding in a patient used as a subject for a long case on account of some other clinical condition. Patients used for examination purposes will usually have varicosities of the long saphenous venous system with readily demonstrable saphenofemoral incompetence. Short saphenous problems and recurrent varicose veins rarely appear in undergraduate exams.

LONG CASE

Here you will be expected to obtain and present a concise history of the relevant symptoms, establish whether there are any predisposing factors and demonstrate an ability to examine the patient.

History

1. Symptoms: ?cosmetic, ?aching or discomfort, typically towards the end of the day or after prolonged standing, ?ankle swelling, ?skin problems (itch, ulceration, etc).
2. Predisposing factors: ?family history, ?pregnancy, ?pelvic obstruction, ?previous DVT.

Examination

Inspection

1. Are there any skin changes (eczema, ulceration, pigmentation, lipodermatosclerosis, etc.)?
2. Which part of the superficial venous system is varicose (long or short saphenous)? In considering the answer to this question, the simplest issue to consider is whether the varicosities extend above the level of the knee? If so it must be the long saphenous system that is affected.
3. If long saphenous, is there a visible varix over the saphenofemoral junction? Is there any evidence of a varix overlying one of the constant medial leg perforators, signifying perforator incompetence? This part of the examination clearly must be done with the patient standing.
4. Are there any scars indicative of previous surgery?
5. Are there any immediately obvious predisposing factors (e.g. pregnancy)?

Specific tests

1. Is there a palpable thrill (or bruit an auscultation) over the saphenofemoral junction when the patient coughs.
2. The definitive clinical test of varicosities is based on the observations of Brodie and Trendelenburg. The affected limb is elevated and the affected varicosities emptied. A tourniquet is then placed around the thigh, with the aim of preventing superficial venous filling from above. It is important at this stage to ensure that the tourniquet is sufficiently tight and that it is placed around the thigh as high as possible, so as to be close to the saphenofemoral junction. If the varicosities are entirely due to saphenofemoral incompetence, a properly applied tourniquet will prevent any filling of the varicosities when the patient stands. Filling from below indicates perforator incompetence and you then have to work your way grad-

ually down the leg, repeating the test until the level of venous incompetence is demonstrated.

OSCE

Patients with varicose veins are common candidates for practical stations in OSCEs. The question may be 'Examine this patients legs' or 'Assess this patient's varicose veins'. In such instances examination should take place in the manner described for the long case above. Less commonly you could be asked to take a history from a standardized patient (as above for the long case patient).

FACTFILE

1. Varicose veins are common. Approximately 10% of the population in westernized countries have significant varicosities.

2. For many patients, concern over varicose veins will be limited to cosmesis. Heaviness and aching, particularly towards the end of the day or after prolonged standing, are the commonest symptoms. Ankle oedema, superficial thrombophlebitis and haemorrhage from a prominent varicosity are other possible presentations. Pain, particularly on exertion, is rarely caused by varicosities.

Discussion Points

1. **Special tests** Doppler ultrasound can be used to confirm saphenofemoral or short saphenous valvular incompetence and can also be used to assess deep vein patency. The combination of Doppler ultrasound with real-time imaging (Duplex scanning) increases the accuracy of localization of venous incompetence. Venography may be necessary in some cases but these invasive inves-

tigations are being increasingly superseded by Duplex scanning.

2. **Treatment**

(a) *Support* Symptomatic relief may be obtained from a properly fitted elastic stocking which is worn during the day and removed at night. Support is particularly useful in cases where other forms of treatment would be contraindicated, e.g. pregnancy and the unfit elderly patient.

(b) *Injection sclerotherapy* This technique is most applicable to minor cosmetic varicosities below the knee or for residual varicosities following surgery. The technique involves injecting the sclerosant (usually either ethanolamine or sodium tetradecyl sulphate (STD)) into the emptied varicosity, then maintaining compression on the leg for 2 to 3 weeks. Problems include skin pigmentation and ulceration if care is not taken to ensure that the injection is intravascular.

(c) *Surgery* The aims of surgery are to correct deep to superficial venous incompetence and to remove unsightly varicosities.

OCCLUSIVE PERIPHERAL VASCULAR DISEASE ★★★

This section is confined to the arterial supply to the legs but many of the symptoms and signs, particularly with respect to acute ischaemia, are equally applicable to the upper limb.

EXAM INCLUSION

Patients with peripheral arterial disease lend themselves to all examination formats. Given the prevalence of vascular disease in westernized societies, such patients commonly appear in undergraduate exams. You will only be asked to demonstrate clinical signs on a patient with chronic arterial disease, as acute ischaemia is a surgical emergency. In the long case setting, however, you may be asked to take a history from and examine a patient who presented with acute ischaemia. Acute ischaemia could also be a focus for discussion at a standardized oral station in an OSCE format.

LONG CASE

Acute Ischaemia ★

Causes

- Acute thrombosis
- Embolism
- Trauma

History

The patient complains of the sudden onset of severe pain, usually with numbness and loss of function of the affected limb. A history of trauma will be self-evident (either an injury to the limb or iatrogenic, e.g. surgery or arteriography/angioplasty). You need to ask about previous symptoms of arterial insufficiency and about possible sources of embolism (valvular heart disease, arrythmias, etc.). A patient with a past history of intermittent claudication who spontaneously develops acute ischaemia with no obvious source of embolism is likely to have suffered an acute thrombotic occlusion. On the other hand, in someone with AF, the diagnosis is much more likely to be embolic. The history should also include a careful systematic enquiry, with particular emphasis on other symptoms of cardiovascular disease and risk factors (smoking, family history, etc.).

Examination

The clinical features of acute ischaemia will not be presented in an examination but you must be aware of them. They can be remembered by the five Ps: Pain, Pallor, Pulselessness, Paraesthesia and Paralysis (sometimes Perishing cold is also included).

In the examination setting clinical examination is concerned with assessing the blood supply to the affected and contralateral limbs (see below under chronic ischaemia) and determining whether there is a possible source of embolus. Full assessment of the entire cardiovascular system should also be performed.

Chronic occlusive arterial disease ★★★★

This is the most common type of vascular disorder you will encounter in examinations. Pain is the predominant symptom and takes one of two forms:

- **Intermittent claudication:** pain on exertion
- **Rest pain:** continuous discomfort.

Surgical Pathology

Occlusive arterial disease is defined as narrowing or complete blockage of major blood vessels, usually as a result of atheroma. With respect to the lower limb, the two most common sites of occlusion are the aortoiliac region and the superficial femoral artery in the thigh. In most patients, a careful history and clinical examination will determine the site of occlusion prior to radiological investigations.

History
• Intermittent claudication ★★★★

Intermittent claudication is typically a cramp-like discomfort precipitated by exertion and relieved by rest. It may be unilateral or bilateral. Blood flow to the limb is adequate for tissue demands at rest but the arterial occlusion precludes the increase in oxygen delivery necessary for the metabolic demands of exercise.

The history should elicit the following:

1. The site of discomfort. Patients with superficial femoral artery occlusion experience calf muscle claudication. Aortoiliac segment involvement leads to buttock claudi-

cation because the blood flow to the gluteal muscles is impaired.

2. The claudication distance, i.e. how far the patient has to walk on a level surface to precipitate pain.

3. Whether the claudication distance is progressive, static or regressive.

4. Whether the patient's symptoms interfere with their life style, in terms either of work or of social activities.

5. Smoking history.

6. General health, particularly with respect to cardiorespiratory disease.

● *Rest pain* ★★★

Whereas intermittent claudication is a relatively benign condition with a low incidence of progression to amputation, rest pain is an aggressive condition with a high rate of limb loss. Many of these patients will already have had surgical or radiological intervention.

The pain is frequently described as gnawing or boring and is often worse in bed at night. Typically, patients learn to get some relief by hanging the affected limb over the edge of the bed towards the floor.

Smoking history and other symptoms of cardiovascular disease (myocardial, cerebrovascular) are important. Analgesic requirements should also be assessed.

Examination

Although the following describes the examination of the legs, it cannot be divorced from examination of the patient as a whole. In particular, the entire cardiovascular system should receive attention.

● *Inspection*

1. Are there any signs of ischaemia (pallor, dry scaly skin, gangrene, ulcers, nail changes, hair loss, muscle wasting, etc.)?

2. Are there any scars suggesting previous arterial surgery?
3. Does the affected limb blanche on elevation (Buerger's test)? An affected limb will also regain its colour more slowly when placed back in the horizontal position and will often become congested with rubor and cyanosis within a few minutes of being placed over the edge of the bed.
4. What is the state of venous filling? Venous guttering on elevation signifies impaired blood flow.
5. Is there any evidence of infection (cellulitis)?

• Palpation

1. Are there any discernable temperature differences between the two limbs?
2. Is there any muscle tenderness (a sign of critical muscle ischaemia)?
3. What pulses are palpable and what is their character? Compare and contrast the femoral, popliteal, posterior tibial and dorsalis pedis pulses on each side.

• Auscultation

Listen for bruits over the major vessels. A systolic bruit indicates a stenosis either at or above the point where the stethoscope is positioned.

FACTFILE

1. Landmarks for palpation of the lower limb pulses
   (a) *Femoral* The external iliac artery continues as the common femoral artery where it passes behind the inguinal ligament. The constant surface marking for this is the midinguinal point, which is half way between the pubic symphysis and the anterior superior iliac spine. A common mistake is to confuse this with the site of the deep inguinal ring, which is at the midpoint of the inguinal ligament.

(b) *Popliteal* Undoubtedly, the popliteal pulse is the one that poses the greatest problem. The most common error is to feel for it too high up in the popliteal fossa where the thick fascia behind the knee joint masks it. The popliteal pulse should be felt at the level of the tibial tuberosity, where the artery lies close to bone between the two heads of the gastrocnemius muscle. The leg must be flexed but relaxed.

(c) *Posterior tibial* Immediately posterior to the medial malleolus.

(d) *Dorsalis pedis* On the dorsum of the foot immediately lateral to the tendon of extensor hallucis longus.

2. Investigations

(a) The ankle brachial pressure index (ABPI) is useful in patients in whom there is doubt as to whether leg pain is related to vascular disease. With the patient lying supine, the systolic BP is measured at the brachial and posterior tibial arteries. In a normal subject this ratio will be 1 and any figure under 1 is suggestive of impairment of the arterial supply to the lower limb. In general terms the ratio will be less than 0.7 in claudicants and less than 0.5 in patients with rest pain.

(b) Treadmill walking tests combined with measurement of ankle pressures are useful in making a functional assessment of the severity of disease in claudicants. This investigation can also determine whether a patient's exercise tolerance is truly impaired by claudication, as opposed to effort dyspnoea or angina.

(c) Colour flow Doppler and duplex scanning can assess stenoses and identify and measure the length of occlusions in larger vessels.

(d) Arteriography is the gold standard investigation and is normally carried out by the Seldinger technique via one of the femoral arteries. Compared with the other investigations, however, it is an invasive procedure and is not without risk (haemorrhage, false aneurysm formation, disruption of atheromatous plaques with acute vessel occlusion or distal embolization, anaphylactic reactions to contrast media, etc.) In general terms, therefore, it is reserved for patients being prepared for surgery.

3. Treatment

The majority of patients with intermittent claudication require no specific treatment. Most patients will improve if they stop smoking and exercise as much as possible to encourage the development of collateral vessels. Intervention is reserved for patients with worsening disease, or those in whom the claudication distance is significantly affecting their life. Rest pain, however, represents limb threat and justifies aggressive management in an attempt to delay or avoid the need for amputation. There are two principal forms of treatment:

(a) *Percutaneous transluminal angioplasty* (*PTA*) This is useful for short stenoses and occlusions (less then 5 cm) in the iliac, common femoral, superficial femoral arteries, and less commonly, the popliteal artery.

(b) *Bypass grafting* The most common grafts performed are a bifurcation (or aortobifemoral graft) for aortoiliac disease and a femoroproximal popliteal graft for superficial femoral artery occlusion. For a bifurcation graft, the patient will have an abdominal scar (either midline or transverse) and bilateral groin scars. For a femoropopliteal graft there will be a unilateral groin incision, a separate scar on the medial aspect of the lower thigh, and usually at least one other scar between the two. Bifurcation grafts are always made of synthetic material, usually Dacron. The best results for femoroproximal popliteal grafting are obtained using the patient's own long saphenous vein.

4. Prevention of reocclusion

Patency rates following PTA or grafting are significantly improved if the patient refrains from smoking. Antiplatelet drugs such as aspirin 75 mg/day also improve the long-term results.

OSCE

Standardized patient

You could be presented with an actor playing the role of a patient who has either suffered acute ischaemia or has chronic arterial insufficiency. The emphasis will be on eliciting the important points from the history, as described above for the long case setting.

Data recognition

Less likely but ABPI data along with other cardiovascular parameters (blood pressure, arrhythmias, lipid levels) could be tied in with patients presenting with symptoms of leg pain on exertion.

Communications station

You could be invited to advise a real or standardized patient with peripheral vascular disease as to the benefits of stopping smoking and/or starting prophylactic measures such as taking aspirin.

Practical examination station

An example here would be 'Examine the peripheral vascular system of this patient's right leg.' Examination should proceed as described in the long case section. This would be similar to a short case in a traditional clinical examination.

Structured oral examination

This could focus either on acute or chronic arterial insufficiency.

ANEURYSMAL ARTERIAL DISEASE ★★

DEFINITIONS

An aneurysm is an abnormal sac which communicates with the lumen of an artery. They can be classified as:

- **True ★★★**   These comprise all layers of the vessel wall and can be saccular or fusiform in shape.
- **False ★★**   Here an abnormal sac communicates with the lumen of the vessel. The 'aneurysm' is not bound by the normal layers of the vessel wall and instead comprises laminated clot and fibrous tissue.
- **Dissecting ★**   In this instance, a breach in the intima of the vessel allows the pressure of the blood flow to dissect the layers of the vessel wall, creating a second channel which may rupture back into the lumen more distally or externally.

LONG CASE

The only type of aneurysm you are likely to encounter in such an examination is one affecting the abdominal aorta (a true aneurysm and usually fusiform).

HISTORY

Patients with such aneuryms may well be asymptomatic, and indeed the presence of an aneurysm may have been an incidental finding on admission for some other purpose. It is likely, however, that in a long case there will be symptoms to elicit. Factors to consider include:

1. *Pain/discomfort*   The most common sites of discomfort associated with abdominal aortic aneurysms are in the back, followed by the left iliac fossa. Usually the discomfort will be low grade and often disturbs the patient most at night. Severe pain is unusual unless the aneurysm ruptures (and is therefore not present in an exam!).

2. *Awareness of swelling/pulsation*   Thin patients in particular may be aware of a visible or palpable abdominal swelling. Establish the duration of the history and whether there has been an increase in size.

3. *Other symptoms of cardiovascular disease*   It is important in all disease affecting the cardiovascular system to consider the overall picture.

4. *Risk factors*   Social issues such as smoking are important here.

5. *Systematic enquiry*   Important in formulating a management plan and in particular in obtaining an impression as to fitness for surgery.

Examination

Abdominal aortic aneurysms are palpable in the epigastrium (the aorta bifurcates just above the level of the umbilicus). It is a characteristic feature of an aneurysm that the pulsation is expansile and it is this feature that differentiates an aneurysm from transmitted pulsation via, for example, a gastric mass. To do this, bring your hands together on either side of the aneurysm and determine whether you are simply feeling the aortic pulsation (transmitted) or if your hands are being 'pushed' apart (expansile).

In estimating the size of the aneurysm, the hands are brought together from either side of the abdomen in the same manner as described above until the expansile pulsation is felt. One to two centimetres usually have to be deducted from the measured distance between the two hands to allow for abdominal wall fat.

Auscultate in the epigastrium to determine if there is a bruit (but take care to exclude the transmitted sound of a cardiac murmur).

As for occlusive arterial disease, the entire cardiovascular system, and in particular distal pulses, should be assessed.

Investigations

- *X-Ray* Calcification within the vessel wall may be seen on a plain abdominal radiograph.
- *Ultrasound* This allows measurements to be made of the aneurysm's size and will usually delineate the upper and lower limits.
- *CT scanning* Gives better definition as to the upper extent of an abdominal aortic aneurysm (intravenous contrast given).
- *Angiography* Rarely required today with the availability of CT scanning but occasionally still employed to determine the relationship of the upper extent of the aneurysm to the renal arteries prior to surgery.

Treatment

Whether elective surgery is contemplated for the patient with an abdominal aortic aneurysm will be determined by:

1. *The size of the aneurysm* The larger an aneurysm, the less the force required to distend it further. Large aneurysms are at risk of rapid expansion and rupture and therefore should be considered for operation. Small asymptomatic aneurysms can be followed by serial clinical and ultrasound examination.
2. *The general health of the patient* The majority of patients with degenerative aortic aneuryms will have generalized arterial disease and are at risk of myocardial and cerebral infarction. In addition, as most patients are smokers, chronic chest disease is common.
3. *The patient's age* Not as important as general health but, although surgeons vary, most will place an upper limit on the age at which they are prepared to operate.

SURGERY

OSCE

The station at which you would be most likely to encounter a patient with an abdominal aortic aneurysm would be a practical station where you would be asked to 'Examine this patient's abdomen.'

A patient with a false aneurysm could also appear in such an examination. These are most commonly encountered in the groins of intravenous drug addicts where the 'trauma' to the femoral artery has been sustained during self-cannulation of the groin vessels. Sepsis with chronic sinus formation is a common accompaniment in such instances. You will almost certainly be given the history but in any case look for the telltale signs of repeated self-injection.

FACTFILE

1. *Pathology*   Aneurysms may be:
   - Congenital, e.g. berry aneurysms on the circle of Willis.
   - Degenerative: this is the most common type and is associated with atheromatous disease.
   - Inflammatory: infection may or may not be present and any vessel may be affected. The best-known examples are syphilitic aneurysms of the thoracic aorta and mycotic aneurysms of subacute bacterial endocarditis.
   - Traumatic: trauma (iatrogenic or otherwise) can lead to damage or weakening of a vessel wall and the creation of either a true or a false aneurysm.
2. *Complications*   These include rupture, thrombosis (with impairment of distal circulation), embolism of contained thrombus and pressure symptoms (e.g. discomfort).

LEG ULCERS ★★★★

DEFINITION

An area of skin breakdown on the lower limb.

Common types are:

- venous (responsible for 70–80%) ★★★★★
- ischaemic (arterial) ★★★★
- traumatic ★★

Infrequent types are:

- Infective ★★★
- Neoplastic ★★★
- Neuropathic ★★★

EXAM INCLUSION

Leg ulcers are most likely to appear as traditional examination short cases or at practical stations (clinical examination) in an OSCE format. As in all instances, however, the clinical scenario can be adapted to other examination formats. A patient with a leg ulcer could be used as a long case, in which instance the focus would not just be on the ulcer but on the entire patient. Examples of this would include the venous ulcer patient with marked varicose veins and the ischaemic ulcer patient in whom you would need to consider the entire cardiovascular system. If this occurred, you would combine the approach outlined below with that described in the relevant sections for varicose veins and peripheral arterial disease. Leg ulcers could also act as a focus for discussion in a structured oral station within an OSCE.

HISTORY

The history of the ulcer itself is self-explanatory and should focus on symptoms from the lesion, the duration, increase in size, and whether there is any history of trauma, etc. before moving on to a systematic enquiry. Diabetes and vascular disease should also be elicited at this stage.

EXAMINATION

Describe the ulcer with respect to its site on the limb, size, nature of the edge, appearance of the base (e.g. slough, granulation tissue, etc.) and presence or absence of surrounding erythema or cellulitis. Pay attention to the appearance of the entire limb. Does the patient have varicose veins? Are there any signs of ischaemia (pallor, hair loss, nail changes, absent pulses, etc.)? Is there evidence to suggest peripheral neuropathy? Are there signs of infection in the limb (cellulitis, lymphangitis)? Remember also to look at other parts of the body, e.g. are the fingers stained from smoking?

FACTFILE

Venous ulcers ★★★★★

1. These are most commonly found overlying or just above the medial malleolus. Often, there will be other skin changes associated with superficial venous hypertension, such as eczema and induration and pigmentation of the skin (lipodermatosclerosis). Significant discomfort is uncommon.

2. Treatment may involve surgery, where feasible, to correct the superficial venous hypertension, and dressings with compression bandages to promote ulcer healing. Elevation of the affected limb is important and requires patient education. Resistant cases may require admission to hospital for enforced bed rest.

3. In long-standing cases, squamous carcinoma can develop at the edge of the ulcer (Marjolin's ulcer).

Arterial (ischaemic) ulcers ★★★★★

1. Most commonly seen on the lateral aspect of the leg, the dorsum of the foot, the toes or the heel.
2. Other signs of peripheral vascular disease will almost certainly be present. This could include gangrene.
3. There may be scars from previous arterial surgery.

Traumatic Ulcers ★★

1. Most frequently occur where there is little tissue between skin and underlying bony prominences (e.g. over malleoli, anterior tibia and the posterior aspect of the heel).
2. Pretibial laceration is a common injury in elderly patients who fall. This injury tends to raise a flap of skin with the base distally. Healing is slow owing to the limited blood supply to this area.

CUTANEOUS LESIONS ★★★★★

DEFINITION

Any abnormality arising from the skin or its adnexae.

Cutaneous abnormalities are too numerous to list in detail and only the common abnormalities likely to appear in examinations will be discussed here. It is important to remember that in the majority of cases the diagnosis can be made on the basis of clinical examination without the need to resort to surgical biopsy.

Cutaneous lesions are most likely to be encountered at a practical OSCE station or as a traditional short case. The topic could, however, be the source of discussion in a structured oral OSCE station. Rarely, you could be presented with a patient with malignant melanoma as a long case.

EXAMINATION

Examination of a cutaneous lesion is no different from examination of an abnormality anywhere else in the body. Palpation is preceded by inspection, during which you should describe the appearances of the lesion, state whether it is solitary or multiple, and mention if there is any other apparent abnormality. Palpation allows you to determine the size of the lesion, its consistency, whether it is well-defined or diffuse, the presence or absence of tenderness, fixity to the skin or deeper structures, etc.

COMMON ABNORMALITIES

Sebaceous cyst ★★★★★

Although not strictly correct, the term sebaceous cyst is usually applied to all cysts arising from pilosebaceous follicles. They are retention cysts, which occur because of blockage of the duct of a sebaceous gland, and are particularly common on the scalp, neck, face and scrotum. The cyst is filled with white/yellow 'cottage cheese' like material which is frequently foul-smelling. A central punctum will always be present, although it can sometimes be difficult to identify. The lesion is 'fixed' to the skin but mobile on the underlying structures. The vast majority can be excised under local anaesthetic.

Lipoma ★★★★★

Lipomas occur anywhere there is fat and are particularly common in the subcutaneous tissue of the trunk and limbs. Because fat is semiliquid at body temperature, they present as soft fluctuant lesions and are usually well-defined, although on occasions they can be diffuse.

Dermoid cyst ★★★

Congenital dermoid cysts occur at sites of embryonic cleavage lines. These are seen most commonly in the midline of the neck, the angles of the orbit, on the abdomen or in the scalp and present as unilocular cystic structures not attached to the skin. Congenital dermoids are lined with squamous epithelium and therefore contain hair follicles, sweat glands and sebaceous glands.

Implantation dermoids are thought to arise from the implantation of epidermal cells beneath the skin at the time of a penetrating injury. They occur most commonly on the hands and fingers and present as a subcutaneous cystic swelling.

Ganglion ★★★★★

Ganglia present as subcutaneous cystic swellings and are seen most frequently on the dorsum of the wrist and less commonly around the ankle and dorsum of the foot. The cyst has a fibrous wall and contains a glairy viscous fluid. Usually they are asymptomatic but occasionally they press on adjacent nerves and cause local discomfort and symptoms in the distribution of the nerve.

Neurofibroma ★★★

Neurofibromas are benign tumours that arise from the neurilemmal sheath and can therefore present anywhere along the course of a peripheral nerve. They usually present in adult life as painless, soft masses and are in many instances asymptomatic, although pressure may produce pain along the distribution of the affected nerve. Neurofibromas can be solitary but the condition of multiple neurofibromatosis (Von Recklinghausen's disease) follows an autosomal dominant pattern of inheritance.

Seborrhoeic keratosis ★★

Seborrhoeic keratoses are common benign skin lesions affecting the middle-aged and elderly. They are most common on areas of skin exposed to sunlight, such as the face, forearms and hands. They are frequently numerous and range considerably in size from a few millimetres up to 2–3 cm. Appearances also vary, from small yellowish spots to large warty plaques. On sebaceous gland areas, they tend to form smooth, dome-shaped swellings with central umbilication containing a keratin plug. Skin tags are probably a form of seborrhoiec keratosis affecting the neck and trunk, predominantly of middle-aged women.

Keratoacanthoma ★★

A benign tumour which originates from pilosebaceous follicles, the keratoacanthoma occurs most frequently on the exposed skin of middle-aged and elderly males. It starts as a skin-coloured or reddish papule which rapidly enlarges over a 4–6-week period to form a smooth nodule 1–2 cm in diameter. Usually there is a central keratin-filled umbilication and some associated telangiectasia. Left alone, the lesion will regress spontaneously over a variable period of time (3–9 months) to leave an irregular, puckered scar.

Papilloma ★★★

Papillomas are benign epidermal tumours which can be pedunculated or sessile and are occasionally pigmented. A variant is the common wart, which is thought to be virally induced.

Basal cell carcinoma ★★★

This is the commonest malignant skin tumour but, although it is locally destructive, it rarely metastasizes. It is most common in fair-skinned individuals who have experienced long-term exposure to sunlight. The majority of lesions occur on the face. Basal cell carcinomas usually begin as a small translucent papule but progresses to central ulceration with a raised, rolled edge. Treatment is either surgical (excision with or without skin grafting) or radiotherapy.

Squamous carcinoma ★★★

Like basal cell carcinoma, this tumour most commonly occurs on the exposed skin of fair individuals but is more aggressive and can metastasize to regional lymph nodes and to further afield. Squamous carcinoma may also develop in irradiated skin and at sites of chronic irritation, e.g. long-standing fistulae, sinuses and varicose ulcers (Marjolin's ulcer). The appearances may vary from an indurated ulcer to a fleshy fungating mass. Treatment may involve combinations of wide local excision, dissection of regional lymph nodes and radiotherapy.

Benign naevi ★★★

Benign naevi are rather variously described in textbooks. The common mole or intradermal naevus has no malignant potential. Melanoma may, however, occasionally develop in a junctional or compound naevus.

Malignant melanoma ★★★

Melanoma is commonest in fair-skinned individuals living in tropical climates but its incidence has been steadily increasing in the UK. It is more common in females, particularly affecting the legs. Melanomas of the trunk, however, are more frequently seen in men.

Macroscopically there are two common forms: superficial spreading and nodular. Superficial spreading melanoma is the variety where a long-standing pigmented lesion changes, for example in size, degree of pigmentation, or symptoms (itch, bleeding, etc.). Nodular melanoma does not arise from a pre-existing lesion but presents simply as a skin nodule. This latter type has a greater tendency for early invasion of the dermis. Remember also that melanoma can develop in the nail bed (subungual melanoma). The primary treatment is surgical and involves wide local excision with or without skin grafting. Amputation of the affected digit is indicated for subungual melanoma. The value of block dissection of regional lymph nodes remains controversial. The prognosis of malignant melanoma is related to the thickness of the primary lesion (Breslow) and to the histological depth of invasion (Clark).

SURGERY

SUPPURATIVE SKIN CONDITIONS

Two common conditions will be mentioned here. Either of them could be encountered at a practical OSCE station or as a short clinical case in a traditional surgical examination.

Pilonidal sinus
Definition
A chronic inflammatory disorder, most commonly seen in the natal cleft and characterized by either single or multiple granulation tissue-lined tracts. The cause is believed to be shed body hair being worked into midline pits where, once implanted, they stimulate a foreign body reaction. Occasionally the condition is seen at other parts of the body, e.g. in hairdressers between the web spaces of the fingers.

History
The patient may present acutely with a pilonidal abscess which requires incision and drainage. In patients who present electively, the most common symptoms are persistent or intermittent discharge of purulent material in the natal cleft with associated local discomfort.

Examination
Look for midline pits, often exhibiting a tuft of hair, and protuberant granulation tissue. Look also for evidence of previous surgery (scars).

Management
Abscesses require incision and drainage. Chronic problems can be managed either conservatively or by surgical excision. Recurrence rates after surgery are disappointingly high.

Hidradenitis suppurativa
Definition
A chronic and recurring suppurative skin condition that affects the apocrine gland areas of the skin, i.e. the axillae, groins and perineum. Symptomatic problems occur most frequently between the ages of 20 and 40 years.

History
In the first instance the patient will usually complain of multiple tender raised erythematous lesions in the affected area. In long-standing cases multiple sinuses develop. Secondary bacterial infection may lead to marked scarring and fibrosis.

Examination
Only the apocrine gland-bearing areas are affected by this condition. Look for evidence of active sepsis and sinus formation. Are there scars from previous surgery? Is the condition localized (e.g. one axilla) or are the other apocrine areas also affected?

Treatment
In the early stages antibiotics are the mainstay of treatment. Acute abscesses may require incision and drainage. Chronic cases with sinus formation require surgical excision; this can range from local excision with primary wound closure to extensive excision necessitating skin grafting.

TOENAILS ★★★★

Problems related to toenails will appear most frequently either in a traditional short case setting or as a practical station in an OSCE ('Examine this patient's left great toenail', etc.) It is possible, however, that a patient with such a problem could also be used in a communications station in an OSCE. In such an instance you might be asked to explain the problem to the patient, outline the options for treatment and discuss the aftercare required to reduce the risk of recurrence.

DEFINITIONS

1. **The ingrown toenail** ★★★★★ This is the most common abnormality. Pressure necrosis between the nail, the nailbed and the edge of the nail sulcus lead to ulceration, inflammation and chronic sepsis. Predisposing factors include tight footwear and cutting the nail too short with a curve at the edges.

2. **The overgrown nail** ★★★★ Proliferation of the nail leads to it becoming elongated, curved and thickened. The appearance of the resulting nail is often described as horn-like. The alternative name for this condition is onychogryphosis.

3. **Nailbed abnormalities** The three most common conditions under this heading are:

   (a) *Subungual haematoma* ★ Here trauma, usually of a crushing nature, results in a tense, painful haematoma underneath the nail.

   (b) *Subungual exostosis* ★★ In this condition there is a small overgrown spicule of bone on the dorsal surface of the distal phalanx, which causes upward pressure on the nail and may lead to deformity.

   (c) *Subungual melanoma* Malignant melanoma can occasionally arise in the nailbed. A pigmented lesion will be visible through the nail. This condition should be considered as a cause for undiagnosed groin node lymphadenopathy.

FACTFILE

1. Treatment of ingrown toenails

   This can be conservative or operative. The former is indicated for mild intermittent symptoms but for persistent pain and infection, surgery is necessary.

   (a) *Conservative* The patient is instructed to cut the nail flush with the end of the toe and avoid trimming it down into the corners. Tucking a small piece of cotton wool along the nail edge can help to separate the nail from the nail sulcus.

   (b) *Operative* The following procedures are amenable to outpatient treatment under local anaesthesia. A ring block is performed in which approximately 10 ml of local anaesthetic (commonly a mix of plain lidocaine (lignocaine) and bupivicaine) is injected down each side of the proximal phalanx. It is important to stress that the local anaesthetic used for a ring block does not contain adrenaline (epinephrine); the digital arteries are end arteries and spasm induced by adrenaline (epinephrine) can lead to tissue loss.

   • Avulsion of the nail: simply involves removing the nail and is essential to allow drainage of pus when infection is present. The nail will regrow but with proper care and attention, as described above, many patients will experience no further trouble. Commonly, therefore, this is recommended as the primary procedure in young patients, particularly if they are female.

   • Nailbed ablation: is indicated for recurrent ingrown toenails to prevent regrowth of the nail. The two principal techniques employed are surgical excision of the part of the nailbed responsible for nail growth or chemical ablation of the nailbed using 80% phenol. With phenol ablation the entire nail can be removed and the bed ablated, or the ablation can be confined to one side of nailbed if only one corner of the nail is involved (wedge excision).

2. Treatment of onychogryphosis
   This is normally treated by avulsion of the entire nail followed by ablation of the nailbed.
3. Treatment of a subungual melanoma
   Following histological confirmation, amputation of the digit is the usual course of action.

STOMAS ★★★★★

DEFINITIONS

A stoma is an artificial opening of the GI tract or the urinary tract on to the surface of the body. All the common stomas are sited on the abdominal wall:

- **Colostomy ★★★★★** An opening of the colon.
- **Ileostomy ★★★★★** An opening of the small bowel.
- **Ileal conduit ★★★** An isolated loop of small bowel into which the ureters are implanted.
- **Urostomy ★** Direct opening of one or both ureters on to the abdominal wall.

Colostomy ★★★★★

This can either be an end colostomy or a loop colostomy. With the former, a single lumen will be apparent, whereas with a loop colostomy both an afferent (coming towards or proximal) and an efferent (going away from or distal) limb will be present, hence the alternative term double-barrelled colostomy. Remember that although any part of the colon can be brought up to the surface of the abdominal wall after surgical mobilization, it is always easier to use either the sigmoid or transverse colon as they are already freely mobile by virtue of having intraperitoneal mesenteries.

In traditional surgical practice, loop colostomies were common procedures and were employed to 'protect' distal anastomoses or in the emergency relief of distal large bowel obstruction. In such instances most are created from transverse colon and are sited in the upper right abdomen, midway between the umbilicus and the costal margin through the rectus abdominis muscle. If recently created (within 10 days or so) a bridge will normally be still in place. This consists of a plastic rod which is placed behind the loop to hold it up to the skin surface. End colostomies are most frequently seen in the left lower abdomen, formed from either the sigmoid or distal descending colon. Such stomas are created as part of abdominoperineal resection of the rectum or Hartmann's procedure. The normal site is midway between the umbilicus and the anterior superior iliac spine, again in the line of the rectus muscle. Remember, however, that although these are the 'normal' sites for colostomies, both loop and end stomas can be created at different sites on the abdominal wall, so always inspect a colostomy carefully.

A colostomy may be created with the intention of it being temporary or permanent. Permanent colostomies are almost always end colostomies. Temporary colostomies are usually loops but may be an end stoma. For example, although the colostomy constructed during Hartmann's procedure is an end stoma, the possibility of later reanastomosis to the rectal stump exists.

Ileostomy ★★★★★

An ileostomy is immediately distinguishable from a colostomy by the fact that the bowel is everted to form a spout which protrudes from the abdominal wall by approximately 2–3 cm. The purpose of the spout is to ensure that the small bowel effluent (which is irritant) passes cleanly into the stoma appliance, thus minimizing skin contact. The colour and consistency of the material in the stoma appliance will also give an indication as to what type of stoma you are dealing with. The usual site for an ileostomy is in the right lower abdominal quadrant but the mobility of the small bowel means that an ileostomy can be brought out with ease on the left side of the abdomen, should this be more suitable for the patient.

In the past, most ileostomies would be end stomas, created after procedures such as total colectomy for IBD; however, loop or split ileostomies are now commonly employed in surgical practice to 'protect' distal anastomoses, whether they be colorectal (after low anterior resection for rectal cancer) or ileoanal (restorative proctocolectomy with ileal pouch formation for IBD).

Ileal conduit ★★★

An ileal conduit is similar in site and appearance to an ileostomy but urine rather than small bowel content will be present in the bag. Usually the bag will have a drainage tap on it so that it can be emptied without having to remove the appliance.

Urostomy ★

Urostomies are more frequently used in children and are uncommon in adults. Their appearance may vary considerably. One ureter may be brought out in the flank, with the other anastomosed to it retroperitoneally. Alternatively, both ureters may be brought out together in the midline of the abdomen, giving a double-barrelled appearance. It is unlikely that you would encounter such a stoma in an undergraduate examination.

LONG CASE

History

Stomas could be encountered in a long case but not as the only point of history or examination which would need to be elicited. For example, an end colostomy will be present in a patient who has undergone abdominoperineal resection for rectal carcinoma. In such an instance, an accurate history of the patient's presenting colorectal symptoms would need to be established. Similar circumstances would be the presence of a loop ileostomy in someone who has undergone surgery for IBD or rectal cancer.

Examination

As for the history, the examination needs to take into account the entire patient and the reasons for the stoma being present. When examining the stoma itself, take into account the features outlined above. In an examination a transparent stoma bag will be fitted to avoid the need to remove the appliance.

OSCE

As 'stand-alone' clinical signs, stomas lend themselves to OSCE stations and to traditional short case examinations. The most commonly encountered scenario would be at a practical station, with an instruction along the lines of 'Examine this patient's abdomen and describe what you see', followed by structured questioning. Stomas and their related issues could also be a focus for discussion in a structured oral examination.

FACTFILE

You may be asked about preoperative preparation of a patient who requires a stoma. It is important that stomas are appropriately sited and that skin creases are avoided to minimize the chances of leakage. Once the site is chosen, it is marked with an indelible pen so that it can be clearly identified in the operating theatre. Factors to be considered when preparing the patient include age, occupation, type of clothing, life style and hobbies (swimming, etc.), and the presence of any physical disabilities which may inhibit self-care of the stoma (e.g. visual impairment, arthritis, etc.). Psychological preparation of the patient and postoperative support are also essential. In most centres, much of this work will be carried out by dedicated stomatherapists.

SURGERY

SURGICAL ASPECTS OF RENAL FAILURE ★★

Occasionally patients from the renal unit may be used in surgical examinations. Many of them will have undergone multiple surgical procedures, some of which are peculiar to haemodialysis or peritoneal dialysis. When they do appear they are most likely to do so within a practical-type OSCE station (perhaps combined with data interpretation, i.e. abnormal electrolytes) or as a traditional short case. Palpable transplanted kidneys occasionally appear as iliac fossa masses in similar settings. Remember, however, that renal failure patients tend to have other problems of surgical (and medical) interest. Diabetes and peripheral vascular disease are common and could lead to such patients being used as long cases.

DEFINITIONS

- **Tenckhoff catheter ★★★** A catheter which is inserted into the peritoneal cavity for the purposes of peritoneal dialysis.
- **Arteriovenous fistula ★★★** A surgically created communication between an artery and a vein, which is required for haemodialysis. The procedure usually involves anastomosing the radial artery to the cephalic vein on the anterior aspect of the distal forearm.
- **Vein loop ★★★** This is an alternative to creating a fistula for vessel access for haemodialysis and may be necessary when previous fistulae have failed. Most commonly the upper long saphenous vein is taken from the leg, tunnelled in the anterior aspect of the forearm and anastomosed to the brachial artery and cephalic vein at the level of the elbow.
- **Gore-tex loop ★★★** The principle of this is identical to the vein loop except that a prosthetic graft is used instead of vein. This may be necessary if the saphenous veins have

previously been removed (varicose vein surgery or previous vascular access procedures) or are unsuitable.

EXAMINATION

Be alert to the possibility of renal failure patients participating in examinations. Those on regular dialysis will usually appear anaemic ('normal' haemoglobins for renal failure patients may be 7–9 g/dl), and many have multiple scars on their forearms and/or abdomen. Patients with functioning transplants are usually of more normal colour but often appear mildly cushingoid, owing to their longstanding immunosuppression. Arteriovenous fistulae will be evident as dilated superficial vessels on the distal forearm (the 'arterialized' vein). If functioning, there will be a palpable thrill and a bruit will be heard if a stethoscope is placed over it. The surgical scar will usually be sited over the anterior and lateral aspects of the distal forearm, signifying the approach to the radial artery. Vein loops and Gore-tex loops are anastomosed to the brachial artery and cephalic veins at the level of the elbow and there will be scars at this level. The loop is tunnelled subcutaneously so that the apex lies on the anterior aspect of the forearm approximately half way between the elbow and the wrist, where there will usually be a further small scar. Function is indicated by a palpable pulse and thrill and an audible bruit. If the patient has a vein loop, there will be a long scar along the anteromedial thigh through which the upper long saphenous vein has been harvested. Tenckhoff catheters are usually made of opaque silicone and pass through the abdominal wall a few centimetres to one side of a small laparotomy incision (either midline or paramedian).

Palpable abdominal abnormalities in renal patients may include polycystic kidneys (very large renal masses) or a transplanted kidney. The latter is felt in one or other iliac fossa underlying a curved scar extending from above the anterior superior iliac spine towards the midline just above the pubic symphysis.

X-RAYS ★★★

You may be asked to look at X-rays relevant to a patient at any stage of a long case clinical examination. In addition, radiology is not uncommonly employed in OSCEs as a data recognition station. Finally, X-rays may be used as an additional short case to fill in time towards the end of a traditional clinical examination.

The following are some of the more commonly encountered films. As a general principle, make sure you let the examiners know what the investigation is before drawing attention to any abnormality you think is apparent.

Barium enema ★★★★

Usually this will be a double-contrast examination – the colon is distended with air and there is a thin coat of barium on the mucosa. The radiologist's catheter may be visible in the rectum.

Pneumoperitoneum ★★★★

The relevant film will usually be an erect CXR rather than an abdominal film. Look for a lucent shadow below the diaphragm, usually most noticeable on the patient's right.

Intestinal obstruction ★★★★

In many instances you will be given two films: a plain (i.e. no contrast) erect and plain supine film of the abdomen. The radiological signs of obstruction are dilated bowel loops (often most apparent on the supine film) and fluid levels (only seen on the erect film). You will be expected to know the radiological differences between small and large bowel obstruction, as follows.

Position
The large bowel (with the exception of the transverse colon) is situated peripherally, whereas the small bowel sits in the centre of the abdomen. Distal small bowel obstruction is often described as a ladder pattern extending from the right iliac fossa up to the left upper quadrant.

Calibre
The colon is broader than the small bowel.

Identifying features
The most important distinguishing radiological features between small and large bowel are the presence of plicae circulares or linea semilunaris in the former and haustrae in the latter. The plicae circulares characteristic of small bowel cross the full width of the bowel lumen, whereas colonic haustrae appear as indentations which do not extent right across the bowel.

Causes
You will be expected to know the common causes of intestinal obstruction:

- small bowel obstruction: adhesions, herniae, caecal carcinoma
- large bowel obstruction: colonic carcinoma until proven otherwise.

Beware the occasional film of distal small bowel obstruction in which the biliary tree in the right upper quadrant is outlined by gas: these appearances are classically those of a gallstone ileus.

ERCP ★★★
The give-away here is that the endoscope will almost always appear on the film, with a fine catheter containing contrast extending from its tip. In most circumstances the abnormal-

ity will be gross, e.g. a markedly dilated common bile duct containing gallstones.

Pneumothorax ★★★

Here you will be given a CXR that may be marked 'expiration', as this shows up a small pneumothorax more readily.

IVU (intravenous urogram) ★★

This investigation can be identified by the fact that there will be contrast in one or both the renal pelvices, and/or ureters and bladder. There should also be a time marked on the film (e.g. 10 min) indicating the time interval between intravenous contrast injection and X-ray exposure.

CENTRAL VENOUS LINES ★★★

Patients used as subject material for long cases may well have central venous lines in situ. Otherwise they could appear in an OSCE or short case examination in which case, after your initial assessment, you could be asked a series of structured questions about indications for and complications of central venous access, etc.

DEFINITION

A technique of venous access in which a catheter is passed percutaneously and manipulated so as to position the tip in either the superior or inferior vena cava.

PURPOSE

A central venous catheter is usually inserted for one of the following reasons:

- to allow measurement of CVP
- to administer TPN
- for high-dose chemotherapy in cancer patients

- to establish venous access in the presence of poor peripheral veins.

SITES OF INSERTION

Most central venous lines are inserted in the upper part of the body to gain access to the superior vena cava. In the majority of instances the line will be inserted into either the internal jugular vein or the subclavian vein. An internal jugular line passes through the skin in the anterior triangle of the neck close to the anterior border of sternomastoid, usually at the level of the thyroid cartilage. This is the usual type of line favoured by anaesthetists. A subclavian line punctures the skin approximately 1 cm below the midpoint of the clavicle and has traditionally been the preferred technique employed by surgeons. Other veins can be used for central venous access, most notably the external jugular. It is also possible to thread a long line proximally from the median basilic vein in the anterior cubital fossa.

FACTFILE

1. Complications of central venous access
   (a) *Infection* The risk of infection is greatest with central venous lines used for TPN. Infection may be obvious, with signs such as pus at the skin entry wound or erythema and tenderness along the line of any subcutaneous tunnel. More commonly, however, the patient has an intermittent spiking pyrexia, often with rigors.
   (b) *Pneumothorax* This is a complication of line insertion and is seen most frequently with subclavian lines
   (c) *Air embolism* Normal central venous pressure is low (0–5 cmH$_2$O – not mmHg) and fluctuates with respiration. It follows that, if a patient is in a sitting or standing position, the effect of gravity means that the relative pressure at the

skin entry wound of either a subclavian or jugular line will be negative (i.e. $0-5\,cmH_2O$ minus the vertical height from the line tip to the skin entry wound). Therefore, if such a line is opened with the patient upright, bleeding does not occur but air will be drawn into the catheter. The patient must therefore be placed supine, or preferably head down, before the connections of a jugular or subclavian line are changed. It is standard practice to have the patient in the Trendelenburg position (head down) for line insertion.

2. Central venous pressure

   This gives an indication of right heart filling pressure and can be used to guide fluid resuscitation, hopefully avoiding the risk of pushing the patient into right heart failure. It must be remembered that CVP measurement gives no indication of left heart function (i.e. systemic cardiac output).

3. Total parenteral nutrition

   The indications for TPN include:

   (a) *Short gut*   e.g. following extensive small bowel resection.

   (b) *Non-functioning gut* e.g. prolonged ileus, mechanical obstruction, severe inflammatory bowel disease.

   (c) *Deliberate gut rest*   e.g. small bowel or pancreatic fistulae, occasionally in severe small bowel inflammatory conditions.

   (d) *Gut unable to cope* e.g. the markedly catabolic patient following major trauma or severe burns.

   (e) *Preoperative and perioperative nutrition* This is often seen as an attractive proposition in a malnourished patient about to undergo major surgery but is of unproven efficacy. It is preferable to supplement nutrional intake using the GI tract (enteral nutrition) if at all possible. For most patients the aim is to give approximately 2000–2500 kcal/day; as a general rule 50% of this will be given as carbohydrate, 30% as 'proteins' and 20% as 'fat'. The major problems associated with TPN relate to catheter sepsis and metabolic upset, e.g. glucose tolerance, deranged liver function.

CHEST DRAINS ★★★

DEFINITION

A tube inserted into the pleural cavity for the purpose of draining air or fluid.

It is not beyond the bounds of possibility that a patient presented as the subject of a long case examination has had a chest drain in situ. Such patients could include trauma victims, where there may be orthopaedic symptoms and signs (e.g. long bone fracture) or abdominal trauma (e.g. postsplenectomy). Usually, however, by the time the patient is well enough to participate in the examination the drain will have been removed. Nevertheless, its presence will come out in the history and may be discussed.

A chest drain may be present in a patient seen as a short case or in an OSCE. In the latter instance it may be part of a data interpretation station, where there would also be TPR charts, blood gas results and radiographs.

INDICATIONS

1. Pneumothorax (air in the pleural space)
2. Haemothorax (blood in the pleural space)
3. Haemopneumothorax (blood and air in the pleural space)
4. Large pleural effusions (to drain these prior to definitive treatment)
5. Following thoracic surgery

FACTFILE

1. *Sites of chest drain insertion* Traditionally, chest drains were inserted in one of two sites: either the second intercostal space in the midclavicular line, or approximately the fifth space in the midaxillary line. Treatment of a pneumothorax requires an

---

apical drain, whereas a haemothorax requires a large-calibre basal drain.

2. *Drain connections* Chest drains must be connected to sealed systems, which prevent air being drawn back into the pleural cavity by the pressure changes that occur during inspiration. Traditional glass bottles have largely given way to disposable underwater seal devices that may have multiple chambers. The principle, however, is the same throughout. The drainage apparatus is a sealed device to which the patient's chest drain is connected by polythene tubing. The outlet of the tubing from the patient is under approximately 5 cm of water. A vent from the air space above the underwater seal allows the pressure within the device to equal atmospheric.

EQUIPMENT ★★★

Certain items have a habit of appearing in surgical examinations. Often this has been as a brief spot test towards the end of a traditional short case clinical examination. There is potential, however, for the same equipment to appear at a data recognition station in an OSCE. You should be familiar with the following items.

Rigid sigmoidoscope

The older instruments are metallic, whereas the modern disposable type is usually made of translucent plastic. Remember that although it is called a sigmoidoscope this is a misnomer: the instrument is used for examination of the rectum.

Proctoscope

Again this can either be metallic or plastic. This instrument is used for examination of the anal canal and very lower part of the rectum. Despite its name it cannot be used to visualize the entire rectum, which is approximately 15 cm in length, compared to the 5 cm of the instrument.

Urinary catheter

This may seem insulting but occasionally simple things like this appear and you are asked questions, once you have correctly identified it, like 'Is this a male or female catheter?' Make sure that know the difference between a long-term Foley catheter (made of silicone and usually blue or green) and one intended for short-term use (made of latex and therefore pale brown).

Sengstaken or Minnesota tube

A traditional exam favourite! In most institutions it will be a four-lumen Minnesota tube you are given. They are usually red, with the gastric and oesophageal balloons being yellow/brown. If you look closely at the opposite end from the balloons you will see that the lumens are labelled, i.e. gastric balloon, oesophageal balloon, oesophageal lumen, gastric lumen. These tubes can be passed by the nasal or oral route and, once in position, the gastric balloon is inflated with approximately 250 ml water. Contrast material is often added to this to allow the balloon to be visualized at X-ray. Traction is then placed on the tube with the intention of compressing the blood vessels feeding the varices, which run from the upper stomach to the lower oesophagus. When required, the oesophageal balloon is inflated using a sphygmomanometer to a pressure of 30–40 mmHg.

Chest drain

Usually this will be an 'Argyle'-type drain which comprises a clear plastic tube, marked in centimetres, with a sharp pointed central metal trocar.

TEMPERATURE CHARTS ★★★

DEFINITION

TPR chart   This stands for **T**emperature, **P**ulse, and **R**espiratory Rate. Often, however, respiratory rate is not marked but blood pressure will be included on the chart. If the patient has had a surgical procedure, sometimes you will see written along the top of the chart Th, 1, 2, 3, etc., signifying the theatre day and subsequent postoperative days.

Temperature charts are another examination favourite. A patient's chart may be discussed during a long case clinical examination. The topic also lends itself to an OSCE format at either data recognition or structured oral examination stations. For example, you could be asked to interpret a chart showing a pyrexia and tachycardia tied in with a clinical history. In a structured oral you could be asked a series of questions about postoperative pyrexia.

FACTFILE

Postoperative pyrexia ★★★

The following should be considered:

1. *Basal atelectasis*   This is the commonest cause of a significant temperature rise on the first postoperative day in elective surgical patients (clearly septic patients who have undergone emergency surgery have other reasons for being pyrexial). It is one of the most common postoperative complications, affecting over 50% of patients in general surgical practice. Basal atelectasis is defined as basal aveolar collapse and arises through a combination of hypoventilation and increased viscous secretion which tends to block the small airways (anaesthetic gases are irritant). The clinical picture may vary from the mere presence of the pyrexia to significant respiratory distress. Treatment comprises analgesia and physiotherapy.

---

2. *Chest infection* An established chest infection may result from untreated atelectasis and usually presents around the third to fourth postoperative day. The early pyrexia fails to resolve but increases, often with an associated tachycardia. Treatment requires physiotherapy, antibiotics and oxygen therapy.

3. *Wound infection* Surgical procedures can be classified as 'clean' (no contamination and no visceral opening, e.g. varicose veins, hernias, breast operation), 'clean contaminated' (opening of a viscus, e.g. GI tract surgery, cholecystectomy and therefore potentially infected) and 'contaminated' (e.g. laparotomy in a patient with a GI tract perforation). In clean operations the causative organism will usually be *Staphylococcus aureus* coming from the patient's skin or the skin or nose of the theatre staff. In the clean contaminated category, the mechanism of infection is blood-borne. A transient bacteraemia occurs on entering the relevant viscus and it therefore follows that the causative organism is dependent on the type of surgery, e.g. coliforms for large bowel surgery. In either case, clinical evidence of infection is unlikely to occur until at least 5–7 days postoperatively. Apart from the pyrexia, symptoms may include wound tenderness, erythema, a purulent discharge or superficial wound dehiscence. Wound infection is an almost inevitable complication in a patient with a frankly contaminated peritoneal cavity, for example following colonic perforation.

4. *Intra-abdominal infection* This may take the form of either a localized collection or generalized peritoneal contamination arising from breakdown of a GI tract anastomosis. In the latter condition, the patient will usually have a constant fever and will exhibit other signs of sepsis. The typical pattern associated with a localized collection (abscess) is a spiking pyrexia. The peaks may reach 40°C, at which point rigors are common. Normal temperatures may be recorded between these

episodes. Remember that the most common sites for intraperitoneal collections are the subphrenic spaces, the subhepatic space and the pelvis. All these areas can be visualized by ultrasound, which is therefore the investigation of choice. Pelvic collections may, however, be palpable at rectal or vaginal examination, while an elevated hemidiaphragm, perhaps with an air–fluid level beneath it or a sympathetic effusion above it, may signify a subphrenic collection, particularly if the patient complains of shoulder tip pain.

5. *Deep venous thrombosis*   This may be associated with a low-grade pyrexia and usually presents at around the tenth postoperative day. Other clinical signs of venous thrombosis may be present.

6. *Urinary tract infection*   Common in all patients undergoing major surgery, UTI tends to be associated with urethral catheterization. This may cause a pyrexia from approximately the third postoperative day onwards.

7. *Thrombophlebitis*   Staphylococcal infections are not uncommon around intravenous cannulae and, if not attended to, can lead to local suppuration and a spreading superficial thrombophlebitis. Venous access sites should therefore always be inspected in a patient with a pyrexia.

PERIOPERATIVE CARE ★★★

DEFINITION

The preoperative preparation and the postoperative care of the surgical patient.

Given that shortly following your clinical finals you will be starting work as a preregistration House Officer, you may be asked in an examination how you would manage a patient at ward level. Any of these topics could appear in a variety of examination formats. Most commonly, however, they would be discussed either as part of a long case or in a structured oral OSCE format.

PREOPERATIVE PREPARATION

You should be familiar with the appropriate preoperative assessment of patients. You should be aware of protocols for the use of the following:

1. ECG.
2. CXR.
3. Blood crossmatching/grouping and saving.
4. Bowel preparation.
5. Antibiotic prophylaxis.
6. Prophylaxis against venous thrombosis
   (a) *General measures*:
     - preoperative weight reduction
     - early postoperative mobilization
     - avoidance of pressure on the legs at the time of surgery
     - graduated compression stockings
     - encouragement to stop smoking
     - stopping oral contraception and HRT for 6 weeks before planned surgery.
   (b) *Specific measures*:
     - anticoagulation using either unfractionated heparin or a low molecular weight preparation
     - intraoperative pneumatic calf compression using specially designed boots
     - intermittent electrical calf muscle stimulation during surgery.
7. Miscellaneous
   (a) *Valvular heart disease* Patients with valvular heart disease require additional antibiotic prophylaxis to minimize the risk of endocarditis.

(b) *Anticoagulant therapy* Patients may be on regular warfarin therapy for a number of reasons, including prosthetic heart valves, AF, previous arterial embolism, or recent venous thrombosis. Clearly the warfarin effect must be reversed to permit safe surgery but, at the same time, a degree of anticoagulation may be essential, particularly in the patient with the prosthetic cardiac valve. In such instances heparin is used; it has a much shorter half-life than warfarin and is therefore more controllable.

POSTOPERATIVE CARE

This may include the following.

Haematology and biochemistry

Patients on intravenous infusions should have their biochemistry checked daily. It is normal practice to check the haemoglobin level the day after major surgery, although the figure on the second postoperative day will often be a more reliable guide as to whether blood transfusion is required.

Analgesia

Adequate analgesia is important, not only on humanitarian grounds but also because it will permit coughing, deep breathing, cooperation with the physiotherapist and early mobilization, all of which help to reduce the risks of pulmonary complications and deep venous thrombosis.

Oxygenation

The majority of patients suffer a degree of respiratory depression postoperatively and supplementary oxygen is required. This is of particular importance in patients with myocardial disease. It should also be considered in patients undergoing colonic resection as the delivery of well-oxygenated blood is important for anastomotic healing.

Fluid balance

Many a preregistration House Officer has been kept out of his or her bed worrying about what fluids to prescribe a patient postoperatively. It is important to emphasize that, in the majority of cases, a central venous line is not necessary and that the key to successful fluid balance lies in clinical assessment, taking into account cardiac function, urine output and the response to a fluid challenge.

If a patient is hypovolaemic, hourly urine volumes will decrease long before there is any significant change in heart rate or BP. Correction of the circulating volume is important, not only for the sake of the kidneys but to restore blood flow to the GI tract where there may be a healing anastomosis. As long as there are no signs of cardiac insufficiency, a fluid challenge, involving the intravenous administration of 200 ml of a colloid solution over 20 minutes, is appropriate. If there is no obvious response and no evidence of cardiac failure, this can be repeated. Assuming normal renal function, once sufficient volume has been given, the urine output will increase. A fall again after a short period of time would indicate that more fluid is required.

A word of caution is necessary. The elderly may not respond immediately to a fluid challenge, even if they are significantly hypovolaemic. If there is no urine output response after infusion of a reasonable amount of colloid, it is reasonable to give a *small* dose of intravenous furosemide (frusemide) (e.g. 20 mg), which may be sufficient to 'kick-start' the kidneys. The danger is that continued infusions of colloid are given while only paying attention to the urine output, until suddenly the patient is pushed into cardiac failure. It goes without saying, therefore, that attention must be paid to the neck veins and auscultation of the chest throughout.

ORTHOPAEDIC CASES ★★★

It is reasonable to expect that orthopaedic cases will appear in the surgical finals from time to time. The following is a summary of some of the more common conditions to expect. It is not intended to be comprehensive and students are advised to consult appropriate orthopaedic textbooks.

PERIPHERAL NERVE INJURIES ★★★

These would most likely be encountered as either a traditional short case of at an OSCE station. This could take the form of either a practical station (e.g. 'This patient is complaining of some weakness and numbness in his right hand – please examine the relevant area'), or a structured oral examination on peripheral nerve injuries.

Radial nerve injury ★★★

The most common injury is fracture of the humerus involving the spiral groove. The nerve damage results in wrist drop owing to paralysis of the extensors of the wrist. Sensation is impaired over the radial half of the dorsum of the hand, although often the sensory impairment can be minimal owing to overlap from the median and ulnar territories.

Median nerve injury ★★★

The median nerve can be damaged by blunt trauma, resulting in fractures around the elbow or wrist, or by lacerations to the forearm. The level at which the damage has occurred will to some extent affect the clinical presentation. With all median nerve injuries there will be sensory loss over the palmar aspect of the thumb and the lateral two and a half fingers. Sensation will also be lost over the dorsum of the distal phalanges of these fingers. There will be weakness and wasting of the muscles of the thenar eminence and the patient will be unable to abduct the thumb from the hand. Opposition of the thumb to the fingers is therefore impeded and the function of the hand significantly impaired. With proximal median nerve injuries, the pronators of the forearm and flexors of the wrist and fingers will be paralysed. The exceptions to this are flexor carpi ulnaris and the medial half of flexor digitorum superficialis, which receive their innervation from the ulnar nerve. The unopposed action of these muscles in such an injury tends to lead to ulnar deviation of the wrist.

Ulnar nerve injury ★★★

Like the median, the ulnar nerve can either be damaged by fractures around the elbow or by lacerations to the forearm or wrist. The paralysis associated with ulnar nerve damage is characteristic as it supplies all the intrinsic muscles of the hand, with the exception of three muscles of the thenar eminence (abductor pollicis brevis, opponens pollicis and flexor pollicis brevis) and the lateral two lumbricals. The hand therefore takes on the 'claw hand' appearance owing to the unopposed action of the long flexors and extensor muscles of the fingers. If the injury is at elbow level, paralysis of flexor carpi ulnaris tends to produce radial deviation of the wrist, and paralysis of the medial half of flexor digitorum superficialis means that clawing of the 4th and 5th fingers tends to be less marked. In terms of sensory loss, the patient will be numb over the palmar aspects of the 5th and medial half of the 4th fingers. On the dorsum, the distribution of the sensory loss can be similar or may extend to the 3rd finger.

Common peroneal nerve injury ★★

The common peroneal or lateral popliteal nerve can be damaged relatively easily where it winds round the neck of the fibula, either by fracture of the bone or by pressure from a tight plaster cast. Paralysis of the ankle and foot dorsiflexors and the peroneal muscles leads to footdrop and inversion, respectively. Sensory loss occurs over the anterior and lateral aspects of the lower leg and foot. Sensation is preserved on the medial side, as this area is innervated by the saphenous nerve.

CARPAL TUNNEL SYNDROME ★★★

Definition

Symptoms secondary to compression of the median nerve where it passes deep to the flexor retinaculum at the wrist. This may present as a traditional short case or at a practical OSCE station.

History

This condition is most common in the middle-aged and elderly or, occasionally, in pregnancy. The symptoms are of tingling and numbness in the hand over the territory supplied by the median nerve (see median nerve injuries above) and weakness of the muscles of the thenar eminence. Often the patient will complain of clumsiness of the hand. The tingling and discomfort are often worst at night.

Examination

May be completely normal. Check for altered sensation over the distribution of the median nerve in the hand, which may be exacerbated by prolonged inflation (1 minute) of a tourniquet to above systolic pressure. Wasting of the thenar eminence is rare. If the diagnosis is in doubt it can be confirmed by nerve conduction studies.

Management

Division of the flexor retinaculum.

HALLUX VALGUS ★★★★

Definition

Lateral deviation of the great toe at the metatarsophalangeal joint. In most instances the first metatarsal is deviated medially, resulting in a large gap between the first two metatarsal heads (metatarsus primus varus).

This may appear as a traditional short case or at a practical OSCE station (or as an incidental finding in a patient used for a long case!).

History and examination

Hallux valgus is seen most frequently in middle-aged and elderly women, in whom the wearing of tight pointed shoes may be relevant. They will usually have been aware of the deformity for many years. After a period of time, a bursa forms over the protruding head of the first metatarsal (the bunion) and this may become inflamed. A later event is the development of osteoarthritis at the metatarsophalangeal joint.

Management

Mild cases require only attention to the bunion and advice on appropriate footwear. If the disability is significant, surgery is indicated.

THE PAINFUL/ARTHRITIC HIP ★★★★

The hip is one of the joints you are more likely to be asked to examine. Students are often unsure of how best to perform the examination (as are many general surgeons!). What is included in this section is intended as a simple guide.

Exam inclusion

A patient with osteoarthritis and who has been admitted for hip replacement is a potential subject for a long case clinical examination. In such an instance, history and examination are both important and must include any comorbidity. Examination of the hip may also appear at a practical OSCE station or as a short case in traditional clinical examinations. You should remember that you could be asked to examine a normal hip in an OSCE or short case setting – there need not be pathology present.

History

The typical patient will be elderly and will experience pain in the groin and the front of the thigh and often also in the knee. The symptoms are aggravated by walking and eased by rest. Stiffness and restriction of movements can lead to functional difficulties, such as in putting on socks and shoes. Symptoms tend to be slowly progressive over time and lead to limping and incapacity. You should enquire about any predisposing conditions, particularly if symptoms have developed at a relatively early age. Such conditions would include trauma/fractures to the hip and Perthes' disease.

As always, in a long case setting, ensure that you take a complete history as, given the age range of patients with arthritic disease, comorbid disease is common.

Examination

Inspection

The patient should be lying supine, exposed except for underwear. First, determine the lie of the legs relative to the pelvis and, if possible, square the pelvis. Look for evidence of scars suggesting previous surgery, sinuses, skin changes or any obvious deformity. Note the soft tissue contours for evidence of muscle wasting.

Palpation

Feel the bony contours for any irregularity; watch the patient's face for evidence of local tenderness. Skin temperature may give an indication of underlying inflammation.

Measurement of leg lengths

Here you need to able to demonstrate and compare the *true* length of each leg and also assess whether there is any apparent or false discrepancy, which arises from sideways tilting of the pelvis. All limb measurements must be performed with the patient's legs placed parallel and as 'square' or perpendicular to the transverse lie of the pelvis as possible:

- 'True Leg Length' This is measured from the anterior superior iliac spine to the medial malleolus. A tape measure is fixed at each of these bony points and the two sides compared.
- 'False Leg Length' This is measured from a fixed midline structure, for example the xiphisternum, to the medial malleolus, and again the two sides compared.

Examination for fixed deformity

Fixed deformities are caused by contraction of muscle groups or of the joint capsule. This may occur in arthritic conditions; the most common deformities are adduction, flexion and lateral rotation:

- *Fixed adduction* This will have already been noticed when trying to place the legs parallel and square to the pelvis. A fixed adduction deformity makes this impossible. If you imagine a horizontal line drawn between the two anterior superior iliac spines (transverse axis of the pelvis) in normal circumstances, a limb can be placed at right angles to it. This cannot be done with fixed adduction and the affected limb will lie at an acute angle to your 'line'.
- *Fixed flexion* This is assessed by the Thomas test. If a patient has a fixed flexion deformity, he or she will compensate for it by arching the spine to allow the affected

limb to lie flat. The spinal arch can be cancelled out by fully flexing the unaffected limb, thus throwing the flexion deformity into light. To do the test, with the affected limb placed flat on the couch assess the degree of lumbar lordosis by using your hand to measure the gap between the patient's lumbar spine and the surface of the couch. If no gap exists, there can be no flexion deformity and you do not need to proceed further. If there is a lordosis, however, the unaffected limb is flexed to its normal limit and then forced further to push the lumbar spine down on to the couch. As this is done, the affected limb will be lifted from the couch and the angle of the deformity can be measured.

- *Fixed rotation*   The rotational position of the hip is judged by orientation of the patella. This should normally point forwards with the hip lying at rest. In the presence of a fixed rotation deformity, the hip cannot be rotated to get the patella into this neutral position.

Range of movements

Flexion, abduction, adduction and rotation are separately assessed and one leg is compared with the other. With flexion and abduction/adduction it is important to discriminate true hip movement from pelvic movements. Therefore, when assessing flexion, one hand moves the limb while the other is placed on the iliac crest to detect any pelvic rotation. Similarly, when testing abduction and adduction, the non-examining hand and forearm are used to bridge the two anterior superior iliac spines to determine if any pelvic tilting is occurring.

Power

Power of all the relevant muscle groups should be tested by assessing strength when contracting against resistance. As always, the two sides should be compared.

Postural instability

The Trendelenburg test is an assessment of the ability of the hip abductors (gluteus medius and minimus) to stabilize the pelvis on the femur. Under normal circumstances, when humans stand on one leg the hip abductors of the weight-bearing side tilt the pelvis to lift the non-weight-bearing leg clear of the ground. If the function of the abductors is impaired, they are unable to tilt the pelvis against body weight and the pelvis will tilt downwards on the side of the lifted leg. In doing this test, always assess the 'normal' side before moving to the affected limb but remember that the limb under test is the weight-bearing side, not the lifted leg.

Gait

Gait should be fully assessed by observing the patient walking.

THE PAINFUL/ARTHRITIC KNEE ★★★★

Proceed in a logical manner similar to that described for examination of the hip. Again, it should be remembered that in OSCE or short case scenarios you could be asked to examine an entirely normal joint: what is being assessed is your knowledge of how to perform the examination in a methodical manner and how to interpret the tests performed.

Typical patients in an undergraduate exam are the younger patient with a meniscal tear and the elderly patient with osteoarthritis. As with the hip, a patient with a painful, restricted knee may be used as a subject for a long case clinical examination. Clinical examination of the knee, perhaps with X-ray interpretation, may also feature at an OSCE station or as a short clinical examination case.

History
Meniscal injuries
Meniscal tears are seen most often in young men, with football injuries being the most common precipitating factor. The medial meniscus is the most commonly traumatized and the usual mechanism is a twisting force to the flexed joint. The typical history is of an obvious injury, as the result of which the patient falls and experiences pain in the anteromedial aspect of the joint. Usually he cannot completely straighten the knee and the next day there will be diffuse swelling. In many instances the acute symptoms and swelling will settle with rest, but when sporting activity is resumed, repeated episodes of the knee 'giving way', with further episodes of pain and swelling, are common.

Osteoarthritis
The knee joint is frequently affected by osteoarthritis. In many instances there will be an obvious precipitating factor. Obesity is the most common but you should enquire about previous injuries and surgery (e.g. meniscectomy). A history of rheumatoid disease or infective arthritis would also be important. Symptoms comprise slowly progressive pain precipitated by activity and restriction of movement.

Examination
Inspection
As described for the hip.

Palpation
As described for the hip.

Measurement of thigh girth
The important factor is the bulk of the quadriceps muscle. Measurements must be taken at exactly the same level on each side in order to make an accurate comparison (measure up from the patella to ensure that this occurs).

Assessment of an effusion

The fluctuation test is the more accurate test of an effusion. One hand is placed over the front of the knee joint with the thumb and index finger extending just beyond the opposite patellar margins. The other hand is used to exert pressure immediately above the patella on the suprapatellar pouch. If fluid is present, fluctuation will be felt between the two hands. The alternative technique is the patellar tap where you try and 'knock' the patella off the surface of the femur but this requires more fluid to be present when compared with the fluctuation test.

Assessment of movement

The only movements at the knee joint are flexion and extension, the range of which can vary considerably from patient to patient. In assessing movement, take note of any discomfort or crepitus.

Assessment of power

As for all other joints, this is measured against resistance, one leg being compared with the other.

Assessment of stability

The stability of the medial and lateral ligaments is tested with the knee in a position just short of full extension. With the knee fully extended, a taut posterior joint capsule may mask ligamentous laxity. With the muscles relaxed, one hand takes the ankle while the other is placed behind the knee. The proximal hand is moved around each side of the joint in turn to stabilize the knee as the distal hand moves the leg to stress the joint.

The cruciate ligaments are tested with the knee flexed to 90° and the foot fixed on the couch (usually by the examiner partially sitting on it). Grip the upper tibia with both hands (which come together posteriorly) and alternately pull and push the upper end of the tibia to determine how much gliding movement occurs between the tibia and the femur. Remember that the anterior cruciate prevents anterior movement of the tibia on the femur, whereas the posterior ligament has the opposite effect.

Rotation tests

McMurray's test is used to test for tears of the menisci and is dependent on the torn part getting caught between the femur and tibia. When the knee is straightened, a loud click accompanied by pain indicates the meniscal tag is being freed. The test involves flexing the knee, rotating the tibia on the femur (laterally then medially), and extending the knee while the tibial rotation is maintained.

Gait

As for the hip joint, analysis of the gait pattern is an important part of assessment of the knee.

TRIGGER FINGER AND TRIGGER THUMB ★★★★

Definition

A common condition of unknown causation that results in thickening of the fibrous flexor sheath at the base of the finger or thumb. The result is narrowing of the mouth of the sheath and swelling of the tendons immediately proximal to it. The swollen part of the tendon can only be forced into the mouth of the sheath when the digit is straightened from the flexed position.

This is most likely to be encountered at a practical OSCE station or as a traditional short case.

Clinical features

The patient usually complains of discomfort at the base of the affected digit and locking of the digit in full flexion, which usually has to be overcome by extending the digit passively with the other hand. Often there will be a palpable nodule at the base of the affected digit, reflecting the swollen part of the tendon.

DUPUYTREN'S CONTRACTURE ★★★

Definition

This condition is caused by thickening and contraction of the palmar aponeurosis. The effect of this is to pull the fingers into flexion at the metacarpophalangeal and the proximal interphalangeal joints. Usually the 4th and 5th fingers are the most obviously affected and the thickened aponeurosis is palpable.

It is most likely to be encountered at a practical OSCE station or as a traditional short case.

Clinical features

The condition is of unknown causation but it is more common in men and exhibits a degree of hereditary predisposition. The incidence is increased in association with alcoholic liver disease. Effective treatment requires surgery, at which the palmar aponeurosis is excised.

GYNAECOLOGY

HISTORY AND EXAMINATION IN GYNAECOLOGY

The summary style for presenting a case is useful in gynaecology. Thus you may wish to present 'Mrs Smith, a 53-year-old insulin-dependent diabetic with postmenopausal bleeding.' This sets the stage and allows the examiners to focus directly on the clinical problem. In certain cases it is appropriate to summarize symptoms in the patient's words. For example, Mrs Smith might complain of 'something coming down', and because you will not have done a vaginal examination you cannot present her as a case of prolapse. General examination is done as in medicine and surgery, although urine testing is often omitted.

Examiners may ask you to demonstrate your technique of abdominal palpation. This is the same as described in the surgical section, although often gynaecologists do not insist on finding a seat or kneeling to be at the same level as the abdomen. The important point here is that, after the standard abdominal palpation technique, gynaecologists often make a point of examining the pelvic organs abdominally with the left hand (standing on the patient's right side).

Many medical schools no longer insist on vaginal examination in the finals. Much more commonly a speculum examination using a model pelvis will form a part of an OSCE station.

You will probably be asked at the end to summarize your history and findings, so do this. Do not repeat the whole story again: this is really annoying and wastes time. As for any clinical exam, only positive points need be mentioned at this stage.

THE CASES

POSTMENOPAUSAL BLEEDING ★★★★
COMMON CAUSES

- Atrophic vaginitis   ★★★
- Hormone replacement treatment   ★★★
- Malignancy of the genital tract   ★★

LONG CASE

History

The important point in taking and presenting the history in a case of PMB is to identify risk factors for carcinoma of the genital tract, and endometrial carcinoma in particular. It is particularly important to obtain/exclude a history of hormone replacement treatment or prolonged episodes of anovulation, as in polycystic ovarian syndrome, and to ask when the last cervical smear was taken.

Because cervical cancer may also present as PMB it is important to avoid becoming too focused on endometrial disease.

Examination

Often there will be no particularly unusual finding at vaginal examination, but comment if the vagina is atrophic (or obviously well oestrogenized). Remember that the majority of women with cervical carcinoma still present with PMB, so comment on the normality or otherwise of the cervix.

OSCE STATION

A case of PMB could arise in an OSCE station as an actor playing the role of woman with the complaint. You will look for features in the history as you would for a long case.

As a communication station you might be asked to describe what investigations are required and how, for example, hysteroscopy might be done.

As a practical station you might be asked to take a cervical smear from a model pelvis.

FACTFILE

1. Only a minority of cases of PMB are actually associated with malignancy. Some workers quote malignancy rates of up to 10% in these women, but this very much reflects referral bias.
2. The vast majority of endometrial carcinomas are adenocarcinoma.
3. Cervical smears will be abnormal in 68% of women with endometrial carcinoma.
4. Age-specific incidence rates for carcinoma of the cervix show a peak at age 68–70, although there is a small peak at 50 years. The majority of cervical cancers therefore present as PMB.

Discussion point

At the undergraduate level the focus in discussion will often be on questions of fact, such as the staging of endometrial cancer and what role staging plays in planning management.

CONTRACEPTION/STERILIZATION ★★★★★

Contraception is such a basic part of gynaecological practice that family planning issues can be introduced as part of the discussion at virtually any stage of a gynaecological examination. In terms of an actual case which might be seen in the clinical examination, however, it is much more likely that an elective admission for sterilization will be seen in a long case. A communication station may form part of an OSCE, an example being: 'This woman requests sterilization. Discuss this with her.'

DEFINITION

Sterilization is an operation the intention of which is permanent, irreversible and reliable contraception.

As a long case this can be difficult to deal with in terms of presentation if there is no other significant history. This may be a problem for you and the examiners to tackle. The important points are the previous method of contraception and why this is no longer acceptable.

EXAMINATION

This is likely to be unremarkable but that does not excuse the lack of a comprehensive examination. Do comment on any laparotomy scars which may make laparoscopy difficult.

FACTFILE

Failure rates per 100 women years, i.e. the number of pregnancies per 100 women using a particular technique for 1 year are:

- **combined oral contraceptive 0.16–0.27**
- **progesterone pill 2–3**
- **intrauterine contraceptive device (second generation) 1.0–1.5**
- **diaphragm 1.9**
- **condom 3.6**
- **Male sterilization 0.02**
- **Female sterilization 0.13.**

Discussion points

1. You should be familiar with which methods of contraception are most suitable for different patients.
2. The precautions that should be observed before prescribing the oral contraceptive pill should be clearly known. You may be invited to discuss how you would manage a woman on the pill, and what observations should be made in the longer term.

MENORRHAGIA ★★★★★

DEFINITION

Heavy regular menstruation.

An alternative definition which might be introduced with benefit here is that of '**normal' menstruation**, which is menstruation occurring in a cycle between 21 and 35 days, lasting between 2 and 7 days and associated with a blood loss of around 40 ml.

Dysfunctional uterine bleeding is defined as excessive menstrual loss in the absence of any clinically identified gynaecological abnormality.

The commoner causes of excessive menstrual loss are:

- dysfunctional uterine bleeding ★★★★★
- pelvic inflammatory disease ★★★★
- endometriosis (including adenomyosis) ★★★★
- fibroid uterus ★★★★★
- endometrial polyps ★★★
- obesity ★★
- anovulation ★★
- hyper/hypothyroidism ★
- endometrial hyperplasia/malignancy ★★
- familial coagulation disorders ★

HISTORY

This may be in the context of an OSCE station with an actor giving the history, or as a long case. The important points are to obtain an adequate history which allows you to describe the pattern of blood loss in terms of volume and duration. A history of treatment for iron deficiency is important, as is one of clotting or flooding, indicating that the plasmin system is overwhelmed. A history of long-term oral contraceptive use is also important, as there are now generations of women who are unaware of what a normal (i.e. non-hormonal) menstrual cycle is like. One of the results of this is that, although sterilization might be associated with changes in uterine and ovarian blood flow and menstrual loss, the commonest reason for a complaint of heavy periods following sterilization is the return of 'genuine' menstruation following cessation of pill use.

Examiners will expect a determined effort at estimating the degree of blood loss and, as above, the presence of passing clots is important. Also useful is the number of sanitary pads/tampons used.

EXAMINATION

General examination is important. You should demonstrate that you are aware of the systemic effects and signs of anaemia. The examiners may not be particularly interested in the cardiovascular findings, but if you find a flow murmur this might be of significance. (**NB**: Do not be too clever. If there is no other clinical evidence of anaemia you might be reporting such a finding in a patient with a haemoglobin of 14 g/dl.)

On vaginal examination you should be thinking of excluding a pelvic abnormality. It is more likely, however, that your patient will be undergoing investigation for dysfunctional uterine bleeding or being admitted for hysteroscopy, hysterectomy or endometrial resection.

If you find an abnormality on vaginal examination think of how this ties in with the history and consider whether it is logical. For example, do not immediately suggest an intrauterine pregnancy with threatened miscarriage in a 45-year-old with regular heavy menses and a bulky uterus. (Adenomyosis or multiple small fibroids are more likely, and the former is only diagnosed by pathological examination of the uterus.)

FACTFILE

1. The average menstrual blood loss in women not receiving hormonal contraception is 33 ml. The 95th centile for menstrual loss is 76 ml.
2. Excessive menses is the commonest cause of anaemia in women in the reproductive age group in the UK.
3. Two-thirds of women with blood loss of 80 ml or more are anaemic.

CHRONIC PELVIC PAIN ★★★★

DEFINITION

There is no standard definition of chronic pelvic pain, although increasingly some clinicians use the phrase to describe pelvic pain when obvious causes such as endometriosis and pelvic inflammatory disease have been excluded. Others use the term to describe the constellation of clinical features that are ascribed to pelvic congestion. There has been a recent recommendation to use the term PPWOP, i.e. pelvic pain without pathology. This has absolutely nothing to commend it.

HISTORY

You are most likely to encounter this as a long case, although structured oral or actor role playing OSCE stations are possible. Often the patient in a long case will have been admitted for laparoscopy, so that when you see her the common causes of pelvic pain will not necessarily have been excluded. There may be a history of previous laparoscopy sufficiently in the distant past to make the clinician repeat it, even if it was negative at the time in terms of finding a cause. Previous laparotomy, including appendicectomy, is worthy of note, and the patient may be able to say if the appendix was actually diseased when removed. The specific features said to be associated with the pelvic congestion type of chronic pelvic pain are of premenstrual ache and 'heaviness' in the pelvis. There is no dyspareunia as such, but typically there is pelvic pain the morning after intercourse.

EXAMINATION

This will usually be unrewarding, but remember to identify any scars, including laparoscopy scars, as some women will forget to mention previous investigations, particularly if the findings were negative. It can be quite embarrassing if the examiner points out the laparoscopy scar which he or she knows about from the patient's notes but which you had missed. If requested, the speculum and vaginal examinations are directed at excluding signs of pelvic disease such as endometriosis.

FACTFILE

1. There are no long-term follow-up data on women who have undergone 'negative laparoscopy' in the evaluation of their chronic pelvic pain.
2. Uterine and ovarian varices have been demonstrated in a high proportion of cases of chronic pelvic pain but there are no control data.
3. Uncomplicated fibroids do not cause pelvic pain.

Discussion point

It has been suggested that medroxyprogesterone acetate improves symptoms in cases of chronic pelvic pain due to so-called varicosities of the pelvic veins, and indeed a randomized controlled trial demonstrated this.

HORMONE REPLACEMENT THERAPY (HRT) ★★★★

HISTORY

You may be presented with a woman (or actor) attending for assessment prior to commencing HRT. Recruiting willing helpers from the menopause clinic is not too difficult.

A history of menopausal symptoms should be sought: in particular you should comment on any vasomotor symptoms, psychological morbidity, psychosexual problems and those related to vaginal dryness, and a history of factors predisposing to osteoporosis, especially a sedentary life style.

You should also make a special point of identifying factors in the history which would make the prescription of HRT controversial, for example a strong family history of breast carcinoma, or genital tract malignancy.

EXAMINATION

This would only be done in a long case. The general examination remains important. Significant observations to comment on are blood pressure, signs of hyperlipidaemia (xanthelasma, corneal arcus). Breast examination, which is important in such cases, is usually omitted in the exam, although you should mention its importance. Similarly, vaginal examination is not usually undertaken in the exam but is important.

FACTFILE

1. The postmenopausal population of the UK is increasing dramatically, and the mean life expectancy for women currently approaching the menopause is to the middle 80s.
2. Unopposed oestrogen in women with an intact uterus is associated with an increase in endometrial carcinoma and should not be used.

Discussion point

The role of menopause clinics is an appropriate topic for discussion, as, for the majority of women, there is as yet no evidence of benefit from such clinics as opposed to the provision of HRT in a general practice setting. The advantages in terms of obtaining long-term research data are very great indeed.

INFERTILITY ★★★★

DEFINITION

Involuntary failure of a couple to conceive after 1 year of regular unprotected sexual intercourse.

Primary infertility is defined as above, but there must have been no previous pregnancy to that couple.

Secondary infertility is defined as above except that an earlier pregnancy (including miscarriage or induced abortion) has occurred.

HISTORY

Essentially there are three possible contributory mechanisms in infertility. The first is failure of adequate sperm production or function. Anovulation is the second likely problem, and, finally, failure of sperm and egg to meet. The extent of previous investigations should be noted.

Investigations into each of these aspects may already have been undertaken, although usually you will be presented with a woman who has been admitted for evaluation, and this is most likely to be laparoscopic hydrotubation. Nevertheless, it is important to establish the likely fertility of the male partner. Another group of patients who are readily recruited are those undergoing reversal of sterilization. The fertility of the male partner is even more important to establish before operation in these women. Thus it is important to establish whether he has been investigated and whether your patient is aware of the result of his semen analysis. In some cases the man will already have fathered children, and this, along with his brief medical history, should be ascertained. Remember a number of drugs – azathioprine, for example – suppress spermatogenesis, and it is a rare coup to obtain such a history if the patient has been admitted for laparoscopy and this is not already known.

A history of irregular painless menses is suggestive of anovulation. The patient may offer a history based on basal body temperature measurements or of treatment with ovulation induction agents (clomifene may have been prescribed in a woman with oligomenorrhoea without prior laparoscopy).

Failure of egg and sperm to meet may be suggested by a history of coital difficulty and frequency (requires tact), or a history of earlier pelvic inflammatory disease or pelvic surgery.

EXAMINATION

In a long case make specific points of examining the visual fields and checking for goitre, lid lag and galactorrhoea. It is very unlikely that you will be presented with a patient who has thyroid dysfunction or a prolactinoma, but these are important negatives and by mentioning them you illustrate to the examiners that you are familiar with the contribution made by these conditions to anovulatory infertility. These should be part of your clinical practice and really should not take too long.

The pattern of hair distribution is also important, and worthy of comment if obviously abnormal. An apparent increase in body or facial hair distribution, however, relates most strongly to ethnic background.

Vaginal examination is usually unremarkable, but make a point of checking that the vaginal tissues are well oestrogenized. Retroversion of the uterus is not a contributor to infertility in the absence of other pelvic disease.

FACTFILE

1. Infertility occurs in 15% of couples. Of these, unexplained infertility occurs in 20–35%.
2. The only proof of ovulation is conception, as the other diagnostic criteria do not exclude defective oocyte release because luteinization may occur in the absence of ovulation and progesterone levels still rise.

Discussion point

Infertility treatment is no longer considered by some health authorities to be worthy of funding. Who should fund this condition if it is 'not a disease'?

PROLAPSE ★★★

HISTORY

The history will probably be of a postmenopausal woman complaining of 'something coming down'. There may of course be a history of incontinence, and this will be dealt with separately. The important points in the history relate to risk factors for uterovaginal prolapse, e.g. high parity, obesity, chronic obstructive pulmonary disease. It is said that women who have been involved in occupations associated with physically demanding work are also at high risk.

It is important to determine the physical fitness of the patient, as this might influence matters towards a conservative management with ring pessaries. Similarly, the patient's home support is important in planning her care.

EXAMINATION

The general physical examination will allow you to consider the patient's fitness for operation, although if she tells you that she has been admitted for operation it might seem arrogant if you decide she is unfit for anaesthesia. Occasionally an abdominal mass is found in association with prolapse, so make a point of excluding this.

The vaginal examination in this situation allows you to illustrate that you are comfortable in assessing this common problem. Do not rush into asking the patient to strain or cough. In older women the vulva may well be atrophic and you may have the opportunity to comment on any abnormalities.

Having examined the external genitalia you can then ask the patient to cough. Make a point of asking her to turn her head away from yourself and the examiners at this point. You can then describe the components of the prolapse and its degree. Examination in the left lateral position using a Sims' speculum should not be omitted.

At the conclusion of the examination you can summarize your findings.

FACTFILE

The failure rate of anterior colporrhaphy is high when the procedure is performed for genuine stress incontinence.

Discussion points

1. The contribution of cystocele to stress incontinence in any individual patient is difficult to assess. Abdominal operations such as colposuspension and use of tension-free vaginal tape have a role even in moderate cystocele.
2. Vaginal hysterectomy is more commonly performed in some parts of the UK than others. Why?

URINARY INCONTINENCE ★★★★

DEFINITION

Urinary incontinence is the involuntary loss of urine.

HISTORY

You may find this topic as an OSCE station with an actor, or as a long case. In either, the aim of your history is to determine the probable underlying pathology. You should by now have met so many women with this problem that you have a well-developed system for history taking. However, things you should pay particular attention to are the pattern of fluid intake, and daytime and nocturnal patterns of micturition. Occasionally you see women with quite amazing patterns of fluid intake who have been admitted for evaluation of incontinence when their addiction to tea would be better treated, so remember and ask. Likewise, particularly in the older woman, determine whether she is receiving treatment with diuretics. You will be used to thinking in terms of genuine stress incontinence and detrusor instability, but remember that physical disability with reduced mobility might unmask incontinence in a woman who would otherwise have no problem.

Determine whether the patient has been admitted for physiotherapy and bladder retraining, or for urodynamic assessment. It is more likely, however, that you will meet a patient who has been admitted for definitive surgery for incontinence. There is a problem here. Anterior colporrhaphy is unfortunately employed by some gynaecologists for the management of stress incontinence. In the presence of significant cystocele this may be worthwhile, but in the absence of prolapse it is associated with a very poor success rate. Try to determine from the history whether there is also a complaint of 'something coming down'.

EXAMINATION

General examination may be rewarding; even in the absence of prolapse there is an association between stress incontinence and smoking, so comment on the respiratory examination.

A vaginal examination, if undertaken, may exclude prolapse. You must try to demonstrate stress incontinence. A word of warning is that in gross cases the urine can fairly splash out, so stand clear enough to avoid ruining your new suit.

FACTFILE

1. Clinical history is only poorly associated with urodynamic findings.
2. Coughing may induce detrusor contractions and give a false impression of stress incontinence.

Discussion point

Physiotherapy appears to benefit some women with bladder instability, but long-term outcomes are poor. Should inpatient bladder retraining be more widely available?

INTERMENSTRUAL BLEEDING/ABNORMAL SMEAR ★★★

DEFINITION

Intermenstrual bleeding is bleeding from the genital tract between menses in a woman with a regular menstrual cycle and who is not on oral contraception (which might be associated with breakthrough bleeding).

There is a variety of definitions of abnormal cervical smears. A practical smear classification, with appropriate recommendations for action when dealing with 'well women' is given below:

Cytology	Action
Unsatisfactory	Repeat smear soon
Negative	Routine 3-yearly recall
Borderline	Treat infection if present and repeat in 3 months or 6 months if there is koilocytosis without dyskaryosis
Positive	Colposcopy

CAUSES

- Cervical polyp   ★★★
- Cervical ectopy/CIN   ★★★
- Cervical carcinoma   ★★
- Endometrial carcinoma   ★★
- Ovulation bleeding   ★
- Oral contraception (properly called breakthrough bleeding, rather than intermenstrual bleeding)   ★
- Endometrial polyps   ★★

Cervical intraepithelial neoplasia ★★★

The associations of CIN are reasonably well established. The specific role of some factors, such as human papilloma virus is well established. Types 16 and 18 in particular have been implicated. Other implicated factors are:

- HSV infection, which may act as a disease initiator
- multiple sexual partners
- cigarette smoking
- young age at first intercourse
- high parity.

HISTORY

Intermenstrual bleeding is a common gynaecological symptom. You may be presented with an asymptomatic woman who has been found at a well woman clinic to have a cervical polyp. As a communication station you may be asked to explain the findings of an abnormal smear to an actor. Finally, improvements in mannequins for teaching mean that you may be asked to take a smear as a practical OSCE station.

As a long case a patient may be admitted or attending for colposcopy or definitive treatment. In obtaining the history, however, it is important to establish whether postcoital or intermenstrual bleeding has been a problem. Establish aetiological factors, although in the examination it is unwise to upset the patient by asking just how many partners she may have had.

EXAMINATION

Often no abnormality will be found on general examination. On vaginal examination you may see an ectopy or polyp but the cervix may appear normal.

FACTFILE

1. Cervical ectopy is the preferred term for erosion, as there is no 'erosive' process, and it is more descriptive of the physiological process.
2. The upper limit of the transformation zone is defined as that area adjoining the lower limit of normal glandular epithelium, and not the upper limit of the squamous epithelium.

Discussion points

1. You should be familiar with the types of therapy available for treating CIN. Large loop excision of the transformation zone permits excision of the abnormal area using cutting/coagulating diathermy and provides a histological specimen.
2. Immunization against HPV is nearing clinical application. You may be asked how this will work in practice.

VAGINAL DISCHARGE ★★★

DEFINITION

There is no standard definition of vaginal discharge, although some textbooks refer to leucorrhoea synonymously with vaginal discharge. Many still reserve this term for a white discharge. A working definition, however, is the complaint of excessive or unpleasant vaginal secretion which may or may not be accompanied by pruritus and/or unpleasant odour.

HISTORY

In a long case the important features are the duration of the symptoms and the exact nature of the problem, i.e. is there an odour or pruritus? A history of previous failed treatment or the use of broad-spectrum antibiotics is important, suggesting the possibility of recurrent candidal vaginitis. The age of the patient is important, as the aetiology of vaginal discharge is closely linked to age. In this regard it is worth mentioning that a blood-stained discharge in postmenopausal women should be considered as post-menopausal bleeding.

In a data interpretation station you may be presented with a photograph of hyphae of candida and asked to iden-tify this and recommend treatment.

CAUSES

- Trichomonal infection   ★★★
- Candidal infection   ★★★
- *Gardnerella vaginalis* infection ★★★
- Atrophic vaginitis/endometritis ★★
- Foreign body   ★
- Herpes vulvovaginitis   ★
- Gonorrhoea   ★

EXAMINATION: LONG CASE

Your general examination is aimed at excluding systemic disease, and you should make a point of excluding anaemia and the possibility of diabetes should, if possible, be further investigated by urinalysis. Often in gynaecology no urine specimen may be available, so mention it if this is the case. In presenting your history it may be worth commenting that your examination would normally include this investigation.

During the vaginal examination you should specifically identify whether there is any evidence of previous bartholinitis (you should always palpate for Bartholin's glands but, as you do in the driving test when you exag-gerate looking in the mirror, this is one situation when you might emphasize this more).

FACTFILE

1. The normal vaginal flora in the reproductive age group is Doderlein's bacillus (lactobacillus), which exists in the relatively acid premenopausal vagina.
2. Ninety-five per cent of candidal infections are caused by *C. albicans* and the remainder by *C. glabrata*.

Discussion points

1. Contact tracing is commonplace within genitourinary medicine, but gynaecologists are awful at this; how might it be achieved in current practice?
2. A proportion of women complain of vaginal discharge when there is no obvious evidence of infection. How should these women be treated?

VULVAL MASS/PRURITUS VULVAE ★

HISTORY

The majority of women who complain of vulval problems will have either a Bartholin's cyst or pruritus. The causes of pruritus have been covered to some extent by the section on vaginal discharge. The other causes usually relate to the vulval epithelial disorders. The history in these cases is usually one of vulval itch in postmenopausal women, although it is also important to exclude – if possible during history taking – other dermatological diseases, including contact dermatitis from the use of biological washing powder for example.

EXAMINATION

General examination should identify systemic disorders such as anaemia.

Care should be taken during the vulval examination to comment on any abnormality in pigmentation.

Any obvious mass should be described appropriately, and it is also important to make a point of examining the inguinal lymph nodes, although this might already have formed part of the general physical examination.

Examine Bartholin's glands and, as the patient is likely to be older, ask her to cough or strain to elicit any signs of uterovaginal prolapse.

FACTFILE

Human papilloma virus genomes have been identified in vulval intraepithelial neoplasia, and the increasing prevalence of this virus may increase the incidence of vulval malignancy.

Discussion points

1. Bartholin's cysts may be seen in clinical examinations, although they are unlikely to remain as the main topic of discussion. Other vulval lesions are relatively uncommon, but discussion is likely to focus on vulval carcinoma.

2. Pruritus vulvae and its diagnosis and management is probably one of the more disheartening cases to be presented with. This is in part related to the fact that the experts (e.g. the International Society for the Study of Vulval Disease) seem to change the classification of vulval disease just when the average gynaecologist thinks they have mastered the previous one. The important point here is that the correct classification includes the term 'vulval epithelial disorders', but many gynaecologists persist in using the term 'vulval dystrophy'.

PELVIC MASS ★★

You may fortuitously be presented with a woman who knows that she has been admitted for investigation of, or operation on, a pelvic mass. The majority of women in this situation will be able to tell you what she has actually been admitted with in more specific terms. Such cases can be presented as short cases, i.e. identify a clinical sign, or as a long case.

Relatively few women with ovarian cysts are available to help 'electively' with clinical examinations. In the majority of cases masses palpable in the pelvis are fibroid uterus or loaded bowel. Other possibilities are of more obscure masses, such as pelvic kidney, which occurs fortuitously in the exam. Beware also the full bladder. The list below is certainly not in any way exhaustive but includes most of the masses you might meet in the gynaecological (and perhaps the surgical) exam.

CAUSES

- Ovarian cyst   ★★★
- Fibroid uterus   ★★★★
- Loaded bowel   ★
- Full bladder   ★
- Pelvic kidney   ★
- Retroperitoneal tumour   ★
- Crohn's disease   ★
- Pelvic abscess   ★

HISTORY

You will be familiar with the likely differences in history that distinguish ovarian cysts from fibroids. One important note is that postmenopausal bleeding is not a feature of leiomyomata. In terms of the other possible diagnoses, an adequate history should be helpful in the majority of cases. Crohn's disease may be seen in gynaecology but the diagnosis is usually reached at laparotomy, often to the gynaecologist's embarrassment.

EXAMINATION

In general, the features of a pelvic mass should be described in the same way as any other lump, i.e. site, size, shape, consistency, tenderness, bruits, percussion findings, etc. The peculiarities of 'gynaecological' lumps include whether they are associated with fluid collections: for example, if presented with an ovarian cyst the possibility of both ascites and pleural effusion should be considered.

FACTFILE

1. The incidence of ovarian cancer is increasing, but there is no evidence that a greater proportion of cases are being diagnosed earlier. The aetiology is still being established, although certain factors are associated with the disease: a strong family history is important and there appear to be certain oncogenes identified with ovarian neoplasia.

2. Staging is important for all malignancies, but this is particularly the case with ovarian disease as newly developed chemotherapeutic regimens must be compared on a like stage basis with current therapy.

3. Fibroids are the most common benign tumours in women and have a significant ethnic distribution, being much commoner in black women than other groups.

Discussion points

1. Screening for ovarian cancer. The observation that ovarian cancer usually presents as stage 3 or 4 disease

has fostered interest in early diagnosis by the application of population screening. This includes detection by routine pelvic examination and by pelvic ultrasonography coupled with biochemical screening for CA125. The success of these strategies remains to be determined, but it is likely that many women with benign disease will be identified and may undergo unnecessary laparotomy. This 'trade-off' has to be compared with the potential benefits of early diagnosis.

2. The staging of ovarian cancer can often be a fruitful starting point for discussions on further treatment.

3. Evidence suggests that the prognosis for ovarian cancer stage for stage is better in women treated in teaching hospitals. Why might this be?

RECURRENT MISCARRIAGE ★★

You are unlikely to be presented with this as a long case but you may be given a printed history of a woman with such a relevant history and asked to outline investigation and treatment as part of a structured oral OSCE, or you may be presented with an actor with such a story.

DEFINITION

Recurrent miscarriage is the occurrence of three or more consecutive spontaneous miscarriages.

HISTORY

It is particularly important to establish the obstetric history in some detail. Depending on the interests and orientation of the clinician, some gynaecologists consider recurrent miscarriage as virtually synonymous with cervical incompetence. There are two main problems with this: the first is that there is no diagnostic test for cervical incompetence, and, second, there is no proven uniformly effective treatment.

A candidate of quality will be readily capable of taking a history in cases of recurrent miscarriage, but for a poorly prepared individual this kind of case can be disastrous, so prepare thoroughly.

The length of gestation at the time of the miscarriage is important, as is the nature of the miscarriage process, e.g. classically, miscarriage due to cervical incompetence is associated with a painless presentation following rupture of the membranes and miscarriage promptly thereafter.

It is important in second-trimester losses to consider the pathological process as being more like the processes of labour, rather than first-trimester loss.

Nevertheless, more attention is now being paid to the genetics and immunology of recurrent miscarriage.

CAUSES

- Idiopathic   ★
- Cervical incompetence   ★
- Lupus inhibitor/antiphospholipid syndrome   ★
- Balanced translocations in parents   ★
- Hypothyroidism   ★
- Uterine abnormalities (Mullerian system)   ★

FACTFILE

1. Of all pregnancies, 0.4% will be third consecutive spontaneous miscarriages.
2. The success rate in terms of 'take-home baby rates' for women with recurrent miscarriage is 68%.
3. There is no proven diagnostic test for cervical incompetence.

Discussion point

Antiphospholipid syndrome is being increasingly recognized as a cause of first- and second-trimester spontaneous miscarriage. Treatment with aspirin and low molecular weight heparins may reduce the loss rate. You could be asked how this might work.

OBSTETRICS

HISTORY AND EXAMINATION IN OBSTETRICS

Obstetric cases are best suited to long cases but occasionally you might simply be asked to examine the abdomen of a pregnant woman.

In long cases candidates often have difficulty presenting the obstetric history, as in many instances there is no 'presenting complaint'. You should know how to take the past obstetric history in detail. This includes specifics about when previous pregnancies ended, how they ended, e.g. miscarriage, term delivery, etc. The mode of delivery and any complications should be specifically enquired about. You may be presented with a patient with a specific problem in pregnancy and who has been admitted. It is important not to concentrate on this alone and miss out previous pregnancies, etc.

Beware one small thing: women who have an antepartum haemorrhage may also have pre-eclampsia, so your approach must take this into account. When presented with such a case it is wise to work out how you might deal with each problem individually and then how you might deal with them in combination. One style for presenting your case is outlined below, with some of the relevant comments. In the obstetric case it is useful to start by stating the patient's name, age, parity and gestation, and the problem. Thus you might say, 'I'd like to introduce Mrs Amanda Jones, who is a 24-year-old para 2 + 0 at 32 weeks' gestation who presented with an antepartum haemorrhage.' People have different opinions on which aspect of the history to present next, and to some extent you can direct things as you wish if you continue smoothly. Since it seems useful to review the current pregnancy, some like to hear the menstrual history at this stage, so you might continue thus: 'The first day of Mrs Jones' last normal menstrual period was the 21st of July 200X. She has a 28-day cycle and she had not recently used hormonal contraception.' Clearly such a sentence must be modified appropriately, but by mentioning the menstrual history you have effortlessly illustrated that you are aware of the important elements. You may mention if the gestational age was obtained from the patient based on an ultrasound examination, and if there was a discrepancy from menstrual dates. An explanation for any discrepancy should be given, as this will avoid an almost inevitable question from the examiners. Gestational age and its calculation is so fundamental that some examiners will dwell considerably on this. If you fumble on presenting such a basic part of the history they may pounce and ask all about Naegele and his rule. You may outline the remainder of the history of the current pregnancy. When you reach the current admission try to include in your history relevant features: for example, if presenting Mrs Jones' case and you are describing bleeding, mention whether it was painful or painless, and an approximation of the volume. Some questions are terribly obvious and it seems a pity to waste your time and that of the examiners by leaving them to ask 'Was the bleeding associated with pain?'

The examiners may choose to interrupt your presentation of either the history or findings on physical examination. You should be able to adjust so that if they ask you to go on to discuss relevant positive aspects you do this efficiently. This does not excuse you from taking a detailed history: some people will focus heavily on the social aspects of a case, and you will be expected to take a comprehensive history even if you do not have to present it. Similarly, when presenting your physical examination you must present the findings on general examination. It is not sufficient to say 'The heart was normal.' You must present as detailed a cardiovascular examination as might be expected of a candidate in the final MB examination in general medicine. In all likelihood you will be more familiar with the working end of a stethoscope than your examiners. Although the examiners may wish you to focus, for example, on the abdominal findings, they will tell you if this is the case. Equally they may wish you to give the results of a full general examination.

If you have omitted something, for example ophthalmoscopy, then say so. It is certainly permissible to say that, although you might have wished to do so, time did not permit adequate examination of the eyes.

Similarly the results of urinalysis should be given.

You will be asked to examine the abdomen for the benefit of the examiners. It is important that you position the patient properly. Make a point of asking her if she is quite comfortable and to tell you if she feels dizzy or nauseated. From these questions the examiners will see that not only are you concerned about your patient's wellbeing, you are also aware of the dangers of supine hypotension syndrome. In this case it is not so much that you are creating a good impression but are not giving a bad one.

It should be impossible to go through your undergraduate training without having to demonstrate your technique of palpation in obstetrics, but do practise this and let someone experienced tutor you before the examination. The rule here is to have an efficient system that will stay with you regardless of the degree of stress you are under. Too many candidates in clinical examinations appear to be touching the abdomen randomly without a systematic approach. Once you have completed your examination you should be able to stop when the relevant information has been obtained. Some people 'poke around' until the examiner interrupts. This does not give a good impression. (In some parts of the world you will find that the style of palpation of the pregnant abdomen is formalized in what are called the Leopold manoeuvres. These consist of answering four questions: What is at the fundus? Where is the fetal back? What is the presenting part? and What is the attitude of the fetus?)

You will be invited to present your findings, and a systematic approach is required. A possible outline, adjustable to different situations, is given below.

'On examination, the abdomen is distended consistent with pregnancy. There are no scars but striae gravidarum and a linea nigra are seen. (Examiners sometimes complain about candidates commenting on such obvious things, but others moan a lot more if you omit them.) The size and shape of the uterus, including the symphysis–fundal height of X centimetres, is consistent/not consistent with the gestational age determined from the first day of the last normal menstrual period. There is a single fetus in a longitudinal lie with a cephalic presentation. The back is to the maternal right and the liquor volume is average. The fetal heart rate is X beats per minute.' This is a comprehensive system for presentation and there are few things it cannot cope with. Additional observations might be commented on. For example, if the abdomen is large for dates it is worth commenting if a fluid thrill is present and on the abdominal girth. Remember that at 40 weeks the girth is usually around 40 inches (100 cm). Suitable alterations need to be made for twins, suspected intrauterine growth restriction, etc. Of course you may meet an examiner who does not believe in measuring fundal height in centimetres, or in listening to the fetal heart. Perhaps you do not believe in these things either, but you should be able to justify your decision. (Think for a moment about why you listen to the fetal heart. Is there any point to it, and if so, what?)

A minor point about your statement about the size of the uterus being consistent with dates deserves mention. Some people use the term 'equal to so many weeks'. It is not possible to determine gestational age on palpation late in pregnancy. If you base your estimate of gestational age on palpation you will never identify a small-for-dates fetus or a macrosomic fetus. Consequently this phrase is sloppy, despite being in common usage.

As in other specialties, try to leave some time to go through your case before the examiners arrive.

THE CASES

MULTIPLE PREGNANCY ★★★★★

HISTORY

Multiple pregnancy could be presented as a clinical sign, 'large for dates' or as a long case.

The vast majority of women with a multiple pregnancy are aware of the fact from early diagnosis by ultrasound. You may be presented with an asymptomatic woman, or alternatively someone admitted with a complication of pregnancy.

The basics of history taking should focus on the relevant facts, i.e. if the presentation is as a result of admission with antepartum haemorrhage then focus initially on this. If the patient is asymptomatic then you may turn early to the issue of the diagnosis of the twin pregnancy.

Multiple pregnancy offers the opportunity to show off the wealth of experience you have acquired in history taking, e.g. women with multiple pregnancies are virtually never entirely asymptomatic, and problems such as heartburn, lethargy, frequency and varicose veins are definitely worthy of comment, but be careful not to overemphasize these.

Increasingly, interest focuses on whether ovulation was induced, and this is particularly the case in women with triplets and other higher-order pregnancies.

EXAMINATION

The general examination should be thorough and, as anaemia is one of the commonest complications of multiple pregnancy, the identification of the relevant clinical signs is important. Remember simple things like checking for varicosities. Do not focus on the question of 'twins' alone. Remember that pre-eclampsia is common in multiple pregnancy, so do not omit to look for the signs of this. Many people will make a point of focusing on the abdominal palpation, and will sometimes try to fit the clinical signs to the knowledge that they already have that the case is, for example, twins. The first sign should be that the uterus is large for dates. The often-quoted way of diagnosing twin pregnancy, i.e. of palpating three fetal poles, is worthy of some attention: in clinical practice polyhydramnios, a complication of monozygotic twinning, will obviously prevent you from identifying three poles, but in fact even with uncomplicated twin pregnancy this can be enormously difficult.

If the uterus is not large for dates then consider the possibility of IUGR, although this cannot readily be diagnosed clinically. Do not be afraid to say that the uterus is not as large as you might expect to find, as you can highlight the difficulties of diagnosing IUGR in twin pregnancy.

FACTFILE

1. The incidence of twin pregnancy, quoted as 1 per 80 pregnancies, is increasing, largely as a result of assisted conception techniques such as ovulation induction, GIFT and IVF.
2. Dichorionicity is not synonymous with dizygosity.
3. The perinatal mortality rate in twin pregnancy is increased between 6 and 10 times that of singletons, and is largely due to the higher rates of fetal abnormality and premature delivery.

DISCUSSION POINT

Almost all of the complications of pregnancy are commoner in multiple pregnancy, so examiners can use this as a springboard to discuss anything from haematinic deficiency to preterm labour. Consequently, you can reasonably expect to be asked anything at all about obstetrics!

NORMAL PREGNANCY ★★★★

Although there are definitions of normal labour there are no widely accepted definitions of normal pregnancy, although most obstetricians know what they think they mean by the term. Those who are given the task of organizing cases for clinical examinations frequently find difficulty in recruiting large numbers of hypertensive diabetics in renal failure at 36 weeks' gestation. This means that there is a distinct possibility of being presented with a woman who appears to be going through an uncomplicated pregnancy. There are a few reasons why such a woman might be helping with the exam. The first is that she is there because of some problem in a previous pregnancy, for example previous caesarean section; second, she may actually have a problem but neither you nor she is aware of it. An example of this might be the woman who has mild anaemia but nobody has told her, and the time that you find out is when the examiner says something like 'and what if I told you that Mrs Jones's haemoglobin is 8.9g%?' The last reason might be that the senior registrar organizing the exam has run out of fascinating cases or they have all gone into labour on the morning of the exam (this happens!).

If presented with an apparently normal pregnancy as a long case your history taking must be even more comprehensive, as the examiners can choose virtually any topic for discussion, and if they are given the information that the patient is 'normal' then they will have high expectations of the quality of the history.

Alternatively, you may be presented with a patient or actor and asked to discuss with them options for example for prenatal diagnosis or for pain relief in labour, etc. Such communications stations are ideal for OSCEs.

EXAMINATION

As with the history taking, in a long case your examination should be fairly comprehensive, but do not forget that you may find a problem that neither the organizers nor the examiners are aware of. Examples might be that you consider the uterus to be small for dates, or that there is a breech presentation. In other words there may be a problem which you are the first to identify, and this is a wonderful opportunity if you grasp it.

DISCUSSION POINTS

1. The expectation by parents that their children will be entirely normal is being made increasingly likely by the increasingly widespread use of prenatal diagnosis techniques. Routine anomaly scanning should be performed at 18–20 weeks, and preferably be preceded by a dating scan in early pregnancy.
2. You should be familiar with the routine pattern of antenatal care in your area.

POST-DATES PREGNANCY ★★★★★
DEFINITION

Pregnancy proceeding to 42 completed weeks' gestation.

HISTORY

This comes back to the importance of accurate dating, therefore the menstrual history is crucial. If the patient is aware of her 'dates', based upon early ultrasound, then these may be used with justification. Accurate dating in early pregnancy reduces the incidence of post-dates pregnancy. One of the worst situations to be presented with is a late booker who is 'past dates', so ensure that even in such a case you obtain as clear an idea of dates as possible.

Clinicians' anxieties about adequate functioning of the placenta mean that your history should try to identify fetal condition by, for example, enquiring about fetal activity.

EXAMINATION

There are no specific features to seek in these cases except to note your clinical impression of liquor volume and fetal size. Clinical identification of macrosomia can be difficult, especially in the obese, who comprise a high-risk group for large fetuses.

FACTFILE

1. Perinatal mortality increases twofold after 42 weeks.
2. The caesarean section rate is also increased twofold after 42 weeks.
3. Meconium staining occurs in 30% of pregnancies beyond 42 weeks.

DISCUSSION POINT

The methods available for inducing labour should be familiar to you, and may well be asked about in discussing post-dates pregnancy.

PRE-ECLAMPSIA ★★★★

DEFINITION

Pre-eclampsia is a condition of unknown aetiology occurring usually in the second half of pregnancy, usually in primigravidas, and characterized by hypertension, proteinuria and oedema.

It is astonishing how a simple question such as 'What is pre-eclampsia?' can upset candidates. Perhaps they are assuming that the examiner wishes to be informed of some of the classifications of hypertension in pregnancy, but let him or her ask this directly.

Similarly some candidates may feel they have to define further every part of the definition, by saying that hypertension is defined as an increase of 30 mmHg in systolic readings over first-trimester systolic readings or 15 mmHg over first-trimester diastolic recordings, or arbitrarily as a BP of 140/90 mmHg.

HISTORY

The important points in the history usually relate to risk factors for pre-eclampsia, and you should exclude points in the history suggestive of possible secondary causes. Previous hypertension experienced when on the oral contraceptive pill is worthy of comment. Family history is also important, given the high incidence of pre-eclampsia in first-degree relatives of women with the condition.

The history of previous pregnancies is important, as the recurrence risk for previous severe pre-eclampsia is between 18 and 25%, far higher even than most obstetricians consider.

EXAMINATION

Almost certainly you will find no significant abnormality on general examination, with the exception perhaps of elevated blood pressure and some evidence of oedema. However, on general examination it is worth identifying secondary signs of hypertension, and in particular it is worth examining the optic fundi. Almost certainly the findings will be unremarkable, but such observations are significant negatives and illustrate for the examiners the thoroughness of your approach. An adequate neurological examination is similarly important and you should take pains to exclude any obvious increase in reflexes, although it is unlikely that you will be presented with such a case. Despite the fact that pretibial oedema is a virtually useless sign in obstetrics, many examiners will insist on you demonstrating your ability to elicit it. There are three sites for testing for oedema around the foot (the dorsum of the foot, behind the medial malleolus and pretibially) and you should be able to demonstrate these.

A thorough examination should not take so much time that you are not able to check the BP and perform a urinalysis. Do not forget the fetal side of the condition, and think carefully about whether the baby is appropriately grown or not. Remember that in some women with essential hypertension (not pre-eclamptics) the fetus is actually well grown, and these women are said to have made good physiological adjustment to their pregnancies.

FACTFILE

1. The incidence of pre-eclampsia varies dramatically depending on the diagnostic criteria used. If one simply uses the definition of a BP of 140/90 mmHg at some time in the second half of pregnancy, then the diagnosis will be made in 25% of primigravidas. If stricter criteria are met, including significant proteinuria, then the incidence is between 5 and 8%.

2. There is substantial evidence to support a genetic disposition to pre-eclampsia, as it is more common among the sisters,

> daughters and mothers of women with the disease, although not among matched controls.
>
> 3. The common causes of maternal death in pre-eclampsia are CVA and haemorrhage.

DISCUSSION POINTS

The classification of hypertension in pregnancy is a topic about which some obstetricians can become quite excited. It is wise to have a clear idea of what is meant by the terms pre-eclampsia, pregnancy-induced hypertension and superimposed pre-eclampsia.

The issue of bed rest is often brought up in discussion of these cases. The actual bed rest is of dubious value, but admission to hospital does allow frequent measurement of BP and urinalysis.

PREVIOUS CAESAREAN SECTION ★★★★★
DEFINITIONS

The definitions which might be used in this context are those of *primary elective caesarean section* and *emergency caesarean* section. The former describes a section undertaken before labour in a woman who has not previously undergone section. Emergency section is a term usually used to describe abdominal delivery undertaken during labour and which may or may not have been preceded by a previous caesarean section. This is not always a useful definition, as a section undertaken at 29 weeks for fulminant pre-eclampsia has clearly been performed in response to an 'emergency', but is often not classified as such.

HISTORY

This is fundamentally an extension of your conventional obstetric history. However, in the context of a previous emergency caesarean section the duration of the labour and the indication for section assume even greater importance. The patient may be able to tell you whether there was a malposition. She should be able to discuss whether she is to be electively 'sectioned' in the current pregnancy.

Previous elective section is most likely to have been performed for a breech presentation, but other factors should be explored.

EXAMINATION

The general examination may well be totally unremarkable but take special note of the patient's height. Do not take her word for it: it is amazing the number of people who are unsure how tall they are. If possible, and if it seems particularly relevant, you might even ask if the height can be checked, as some women will claim to be quite different from the height recorded in the notes the examiners will have access to.

Obviously on abdominal palpation there will be a scar, but it is remarkably easy to report your findings and forget to mention it, particularly if a Pfannenstiel incision has been used. Beware commenting on whether a caesarean section was 'classic' or not. Midline incisions used to be commonly used for all abdominal deliveries, and consequently most such incisions were used for lower-segment operations as well as classic operations.

FACTFILE

1. The caesarean section rate in the UK is rising and the major contributing factors are dystocia (failure to progress), presumed fetal distress (without fetal blood sampling) and previous caesarean section. 'Failure to progress' is not a diagnosis and most cases of caesarean section will result from poorly managed malposition or dysfunctional labour in a primigravida.

2. Uterine rupture occurs in 1.5% of previous caesarean sections and is approximately 19 times more common following classic section compared with the lower segment operation.

DISCUSSION POINTS

1. The selected method of delivery in a woman with a previous section provides the usual topic for discussion and you should be prepared to talk about what factors would influence you toward or away from vaginal delivery.

2. The high section rate and methods of reducing this are fair topics which indicate the clinical exposure of the candidate.

SMALL FOR DATES ★★★★

DEFINITION

A fetus which is below an arbitrary centile value of weight for gestational age. Some centres use the 10th centile, but an increasing number use the fifth centile and some the third. The third centile identifies a subset which more accurately pinpoints fetuses likely to be genuinely growth restricted in utero as well as SFD. It is worth making a small point here: the term growth 'restriction' is increasingly being used in place of the more usual growth 'retardation'. 'Restriction' should be the preferred term, not only because it more actually describes the pathophysiology but also because its use is preferable to parents, for whom the term retardation may have other alarming associations.

It is important to distinguish clearly between IUGR and being SFD. Failure of a fetus 'to meet its genetically determined growth velocity' is the prime feature of IUGR, but not one that can be recognized clinically.

Cases may be recognized by observing a reduction in fetal growth velocity, as evidenced by serial ultrasound measurements, but in clinical practice as well as the clinical examination you are more likely to be presented with a clinically SFD fetus. (It is important to appreciate that from the definition of IUGR a fetus need not be SFD to be suffering growth restriction, but this is a concept with which many clinicians are uncomfortable.)

CAUSES

- Wrong dates   ★★★
- IUGR   ★★★★★
- Constitutional   ★★★★★
- Ethnic   ★★★
- Fetal anomaly   ★★
- Maternal smoking   ★★★
- Drug misuse   ★★
- Fetal infection   ★
- Pre-eclampsia   ★★★★
- Previous SFD   ★★★★★

You may see a case of SFD as a clinical sign in an OSCE station or as a long case.

HISTORY

Many of the women who are thought to be SFD will be recruited to the examination either while they are inpatients admitted for evaluation or attending a day unit for fetal assessment. Consequently, most will be aware that there may be a problem with fetal growth or wellbeing.

It is important not to be side-tracked by the immediate issue of evaluating the fetus: the important point is to establish whether the fetus is actually SFD. The first issue, therefore, is whether the dates are accurate. Some examiners will focus very heavily indeed on menstrual data. You must establish the gestational age from dates as reliably as possible, and if there is doubt about the dates any additional information is essential. Clearly many women will be aware of the gestational age derived from an ultrasound examination. You should be aware of the likely accuracy of ultrasound estimation of gestational age, as in women who book late in the second trimester ultrasound is not much more help in dating than a history of when quickening was noted.

The past obstetric history is one of the most important parts of the history, as the single largest risk factor for the delivery of an SFD fetus is a previous event. Social history is very important insofar as it is known that smoking and drug misuse are associated with SFD fetuses.

EXAMINATION

General examination is designed to identify potential causes of SFD and possibly IUGR. Comment on physical evidence suggesting heavy smoking or evidence of chronic disease.

The main issue by the time you come to examine the abdomen will be whether fetal size is consistent with the gestational age you have arrived at. You must ask yourself if the uterus really is SFD. The clinical signs associated with IUGR are that the uterus is SFD, the fetus feels flexed, the liquor volume feels reduced and the fetal parts are more readily felt.

FACTFILE

Recognition of the SFD fetus is notoriously difficult and this might lead some people to a sense of nihilism, as only 50% of SFD fetuses are actually identified as such. This relatively poor sensitivity in detection is matched by the fact that, of every three fetuses suspected of being SFD, only one actually is.

DISCUSSION POINT

The most frequent problems in the management of suspected SFD cases are the resolution of the accuracy of gestational age assessment, the question of when to deliver, and how to evaluate fetal wellbeing before this. Most evaluation is based on biophysical assessment, particularly cardiotocography.

ANTEPARTUM HAEMORRHAGE ★★★

DEFINITION

Bleeding from the genital tract from 24 weeks' gestation to delivery.

CAUSES

- Placenta praevia ★★★ A condition wherein the placenta or a part thereof lies in the lower uterine segment (the lower uterine segment is that part of the uterus which lies below the reflection of the uterovesical peritoneum).
- Placental abruption ★★ A condition in which a normally sited placenta separates prematurely from the uterine wall.
- Marginal haemorrhage ★★★
- Cervical polyp/polyp ★★
- Cervical carcinoma ★
- Spurious causes include haematuria and rectal bleeding

HISTORY

When you are presented with a woman who gives a history of vaginal bleeding the important features are: when the bleeding occurred, an estimate of the volume, whether it was associated with abdominal pain and whether it was postcoital.

Repeated episodes of bleeding are a feature of placenta praevia, so be careful when you ask when the bleeding occurred: you may find the patient tells you about the most recent event, and not any earlier episodes. Clinicians' estimates of vaginal bleeding are pretty awful and patients themselves are not particularly good, as to an anxious woman a small volume may look like major haemorrhage. Bleeding which is heavier or lighter than a period is a useful distinction, as the woman at least has a reference point. A history such as 'the bed was soaked' is useful, but most women whose pregnancies get to the stage of helping with examinations will have a history of lighter bleeding, and you might ask if the blood soaked through her underwear or not. These are more useful reference points than asking someone to estimate if the volume lost was equivalent to a cupful, etc. Painful bleeding is said to identify abruption rather than placenta praevia, but if a woman is in preterm labour she may complain of painful contractions while bleeding from a low-lying placenta. Tactful enquiry about whether the bleeding was postcoital is worthwhile, and may even be a significant negative.

When taking the history in the examination setting it is understood that further investigations might have been performed; for example, you may reasonably ask the patient whether she is aware of the site of the placenta from a previous ultrasound scan.

It is also worth asking the patient about findings from earlier investigation; in particular, did she have a cervical smear in the recent past, and if so does she know the result?

EXAMINATION

It is important to confirm on general examination that there is no evidence of anaemia or other sign of recent significant blood loss. Hypertension is a more likely finding than being presented with a hypotensive shocked woman!

On abdominal palpation you should try to identify pointers towards or away from a diagnosis of placenta praevia: clearly a transverse lie or very high presenting part are suggestive, but do not forget that your patient may be having recurrent small abruptions and consider that the uterus might be small for dates. In other words, remember that other diagnoses should be considered. The examiners might be fed up hearing about antepartum haemorrhage and be looking for something else to discuss.

It is unlikely that you will meet a woman in the examination with a tense hard abdomen and absent fetal heart, but you should be prepared to discuss the findings you would anticipate in severe abruption.

FACTFILE

1. APH complicates 2–4% of pregnancies.
2. Performing a vaginal examination in a woman presenting with APH without either prior (reliable) knowledge of the placental site or outwith an operating theatre with facilities for immediate delivery is dangerous. Do not let an examiner try to talk you into saying that the clinical diagnosis of abruption is so easy that you should go ahead and rupture the membranes in the ordinary delivery room.

Discussion point

It is very easy to confuse candidates about the management of placenta praevia, particularly when some talk about EUA (examination under anaesthesia) and EWA (examination without anaesthetic). These confusing terms might indicate that examination is performed under anaesthetic or without anaesthetic, respectively, but remember that 'with' and 'without' both begin with W, and the conservative management of placenta praevia is so very well defined that you should be familiar with its principles. The availability of placentography has, of course, changed the approach to the management of APH, but the clinical examination setting tests knowledge of basic principles as much as knowledge of new techniques.

BREECH PRESENTATION ★★★★

DEFINITION

Breech presentation is pretty much self-explanatory, but you must be able to define the types of breech presentation. *Flexed breech* is a breech presentation with flexion at knees and hips. *Frank breech* describes flexion at the hip and extension at the knees. *Footling presentation* is said to be an incomplete breech presentation, i.e. one or both feet or knee(s) presents.

HISTORY

You may be presented with a patient who is attending to help with the examination purely because of a breech presentation (in which case part of her history will address this specifically), or breech presentation may be incidental to her attendance either to help with the examination or for routine antenatal care. In this case she may not mention the fact of breech presentation (or even be aware of it). As the incidence of breech presentation is closely related to gestational age, the earlier the gestation of any patient you see, the greater the chance of finding a breech presentation. Remember that a case of pre-eclampsia may still also be complicated by a breech presentation, but it is worth analysing your management of each of these problems individually before amalgamating your approach for the more complex situation.

Try to identify or exclude factors leading to breech presentation: high parity, abnormal uterine shape and multiple pregnancy are always mentioned in the textbooks, but in the majority of women there will not be much in the way of specific facts in the history.

The undoubted association with fetal anomaly is important, and a history of satisfactory detailed ultrasound examination is reassuring. Placentography may have been performed, and it is worth asking if the patient knows whether or not this has been done.

EXAMINATION

One of the more reassuring comments in one of the standard textbooks is that there is no characteristic finding on abdominal palpation. The point of this is that if on palpation the diagnosis is not too obvious, it is no crime to say so.

The clinical features of breech presentation need not be rehearsed here except to mention that occasionally in a cephalic presentation the breech will be ballotable in the fundus, and this can be confusing because some think that a ballotable pole in the fundus must be the head. Secondly, even if you think the fetal head is well down in a cephalic presentation, beware missing a breech presentation, which can feel very similar to a well-engaged head on abdominal palpation. The final thing to say about examination of a presumed breech presentation is that just because a woman is kind enough to agree to help with the examination when she has been seen at the antenatal clinic the week before, this does not preclude the possibility of spontaneous version. Consequently, if you are certain she has a cephalic presentation then say so.

FACTFILE

Breech presentation occurs in 3% of deliveries at term, but is found in 28% of pregnancies at 28 weeks' gestation and 10% at 32 weeks.

DISCUSSION POINTS

1. The principal areas of controversy relate to the value of external cephalic version and the mode of delivery.

2. The contraindications to version can also provoke interesting discussion. The list usually given is: planned caesarean section, previous caesarean section, multiple pregnancy, placenta praevia and fetal abnormality.

LARGE FOR DATES ★★★

Unlike the term 'small for dates' there is no standard definition of large for dates. A functional definition might be that the uterus is large for dates if uterine size is greater than might normally be expected for the given gestation.

Macrosomia is the term used to describe a fetus which is above an arbitrary fetal weight. In North American textbooks macrosomia is used to describe fetuses weighing 4 kg or more. In British practice a 4.5 kg cut-off point is more commonly used.

Causes

- Wrong dates   ★★★
- Multiple pregnancy   ★★★★
- Macrosomic fetus (including diabetic
  pregnancy)   ★★★
- Gravid fibroid uterus   ★★
- Polyhydramnios   ★★★★

POLYHYDRAMNIOS

This term describes excessive liquor volume. Again there is no standard definition of polyhydramnios, but the term is used widely to describe the situation where the liquor volume is thought to be excessive. Liquor volume varies markedly with gestation, and even within a single gestational age there is a wide variation.

This will most commonly present as a clinical sign station.

CAUSES

- Idiopathic   ★★★★
- Anencephaly   ★
- Open spina bifida   ★
- Gastroschisis   ★
- Exomphalos   ★
- Oesophageal atresia   ★★
- Duodenal atresia   ★★★
- Monozygotic twin pregnancy   ★★
- Diabetes   ★★★

HISTORY

The importance of gestational age and its calculation is as relevant here as in the small-for-dates fetus.

The history in cases of polyhydramnios is variable: the patient may be aware that she is thought to be large but be asymptomatic. The history in symptomatic polyhydramnios is usually of a relatively acute increase in uterine size. This might present with the patient actually complaining of a feeling of her skin being stretched, or with marked oesophageal reflux or worsening haemorrhoids or varicose veins.

You should be able to determine from the patient which investigations have already been performed and identify which of the possible causes have probably already been excluded.

EXAMINATION

General examination in cases of polyhydramnios will confirm peripheral oedema and allow you to identify lower limb varices.

On abdominal palpation the important thing is to identify whether the uterus is actually large for dates. The important points are to determine which of the uterine contents are present excessively and, having done so, be logical in your presentation. It is difficult to take seriously a candidate who says that the liquor volume is markedly increased but that the fetal parts are easily felt and the fetal heart readily heard, etc.

The fundal height should be measured in centimetres, and traditionally the abdominal girth in inches. Try to elicit a fluid thrill.

DISCUSSION POINTS

1. The differential diagnosis of large for dates is interesting because the exclusion of the commoner diagnoses covers many areas of obstetrics, from gestational diabetes to screening for neural tube defect.
2. The importance of diagnosing the macrosomic fetus is much less emphasized in British obstetric practice than in American, but the importation of the same attitudes to litigation may result in an increasing focus on this. The background to this is the higher incidence of shoulder dystocia.

MEDICAL DISORDERS IN PREGNANCY (excluding diabetes)
★★★

The approach to medical disorders in pregnancy should address two areas: the effect of the disease on the pregnancy and the effect of the pregnancy on the disease.

The more common disorders you are likely to meet are:

- epilepsy   ★★★★
- hyperthyroidism   ★★
- asthma   ★★★★
- cardiac disease (usually asymptomatic)   ★★
- essential hypertension   ★★★
- anaemias (including haemoglobinopathies)   ★★★

Epilepsy and its interaction with pregnancy exemplifies the value of a logical approach to the resultant problems. The effect of epilepsy on pregnancy is mediated by both the disease and its treatment. Presumed hypoxic episodes during grand mal seizures may play some role in the higher incidence of fetal anomalies seen in the infants of epileptics. This higher incidence of fetal abnormality is a feature of the disease, rather than the drugs used in treatment. Nevertheless, it is likely that all drugs used in the management of epilepsy are teratogenic to some extent: sodium valproate and phenytoin are always mentioned in this regard, but even carbamazepine is now recognized as causing some malformations. Sodium valproate has a significant association with neural tube defect.

Pregnancy has a variable effect on the frequency of convulsions, although, when this worsens, management problems are compounded by the difficulty of monitoring therapeutic levels in pregnancy.

Epilepsy is also the paradigm for prepregnancy rationalization of treatment because reduction in the dosage or number of anticonvulsants will reduce the risk of malformation. In women with idiopathic epilepsy it may be possible to stop therapy in early pregnancy if the patient has been fit-free for 2 or more years.

Essential hypertension merits further mention, as the effect of mild or moderate hypertension in pregnancy is probably not particularly adverse. The value of treating moderate hypertension in pregnancy is not proven. Atenolol, if given from early in the second trimester, is associated with IUGR and fetal death. Methyldopa appears to be safe throughout pregnancy and has the merit of long-term follow-up data. Pre-eclampsia superimposed on essential hypertension is bad news, but there is no evidence that lowering blood pressure in early pregnancy reduces the risk of this developing.

Finally, anaemia is yet another area where some obstetricians will expect you to be able to discuss the physiology of iron and folate metabolism at length.

In cosmopolitan areas there is a distinct possibility of meeting a patient with one of the haemoglobinopathies. This affords you the possibility of showing off your knowledge of the effect of the disease on the pregnancy, with particular regard to the role of prenatal diagnosis. If your examiner is not from an area of large immigrant populations then your knowledge of the genetics of the thalassaemias could impress!

Deep venous thrombosis is clinically very important and its exclusion may be relevant in any of your gynaecological or obstetrical cases. Obtain a detailed history of the previous event. A family history may be important: the contribution of deficiencies in antithrombin III, protein C, protein S and the presence of factor V Leiden is being increasingly recognized.

EXAMINATION

The important point is to elicit the physical signs pertinent to the underlying medical disorder.

PRETERM PREMATURE RUPTURE OF THE MEMBRANES
★★★

DEFINITION

Rupture of the membranes without establishment of labour before 37 weeks' gestation.

NB: There is considerable confusion about the meaning of premature rupture of the membranes. Without the prefix 'preterm', this is used in North America to describe rupture of the membranes before labour is established, regardless of the gestational age.

HISTORY

The history in cases of suspected rupture of the membranes is usually straightforward: the patient complains of leaking fluid vaginally. This may have begun in a gush of fluid or, alternatively, with a continuous leak of small volumes of fluid. The likeliest source of confusion is with urinary incontinence, which is common in pregnancy. The gestation at which the membranes ruptured and the duration of PPROM should be established. You should try to exclude the more serious sequelae of PPROM, particularly chorionamnionitis. A history of flu-like illness should therefore be elicited if possible.

Check whether a speculum examination was performed and whether any bacteriological swabs were taken to exclude infection. Similarly, it may be that liquor was collected for measurement of the lecithin/sphingomyelin ratio and the identification of phosphatidyl glycerol. Clearly not all women would be able to tell you what investigations might have been performed, but do ask.

Similarly you might try to elicit a history of whether steroids were administered to accelerate fetal lung maturity. If rupture of the membranes occurs at term and your patient has been recruited to help with the exam, then she will probably be able to tell you whether a plan to induce labour has been decided upon.

EXAMINATION

On general examination you need to exclude signs of infection, particularly tachycardia and pyrexia. The absence of such signs is worthy of comment.

On abdominal examination exclude uterine tenderness and comment on any reduction in liquor which is clinically obvious. Remember that just because you think the liquor volume should be reduced in cases of PPROM, this does not mean that it will be clinically apparent. If you think the liquor volume is normal then have the courage to say so.

OBSTETRICS

FACTFILE

1. The processes leading to rupture of the membranes are incompletely understood, but it is known that the collagen content of amnion reduces towards term.
2. *Escherichia coli, Bacteroides fragilis* infection and the presence of beta-haemolytic streptococci have been found in association with PPROM, but their role in rupturing the membranes is unknown.

DISCUSSION POINTS

1. You will be expected to be familiar with the policy relating to the use of steroids to accelerate fetal lung maturity.
2. PPROM lends itself to discussion on what factors influence the onset of labour.

PREVIOUS POSTPARTUM HAEMORRHAGE ★★

DEFINITION

Primary PPH is defined as vaginal bleeding of 500 ml or more within 24 hours of delivery. *Secondary* PPH is not quantified by volume, but is 'excessive' vaginal bleeding more than 24 hours after delivery until 6 weeks postpartum.

You may meet an actor who, as part of a communication station, will give a history of PPH. Alternatively you may meet a woman in a normal pregnancy who gives such a history in a long case.

CAUSES

- Atonic uterus ★
- Retained placenta /placental part ★★
- Trauma, particularly cervical ★★

HISTORY

If the only abnormality you have detected in the history is of a previous PPH then the likelihood is that the current pregnancy is normal. Alternatively, there is something you have missed but do not panic.

The important parts of the history to determine are: when the bleeding occurred in relation to delivery; whether the patient became 'unwell'; whether blood transfusion was required; and finally, whether examination was undertaken in theatre.

FACTFILE

1. PPH is the most common cause of severe hypotension in obstetric practice.
2. Prolonged labour, multiple pregnancy and polyhydramnios are all associated with PPH, but the commonest cause, as it is invariably associated with loss of more than 500 ml, is caesarean section.

DISCUSSION POINTS

1. The normal management of the third stage of labour is a favourite question for students. Similarly, knowledge of the pharmacology of ergometrine and oxytocin is essential, as is how a case of primary PPH should be managed.
2. You may be asked how the third stage should be managed in the current pregnancy. This will be influenced by the aetiology of the problem in the last pregnancy.

DIABETES IN PREGNANCY ★

DEFINITION

A clinical syndrome characterized by hyperglycaemia caused by relative insulin deficiency or reduced effectiveness of insulin.

The more recent classifications of diabetes into type 1 and type 2 disease may be unknown to some examiners, who are more familiar with the terms insulin dependent and non-insulin dependent. Gestational diabetes is defined as diabetes developing during pregnancy and resolving after delivery.

HISTORY

The main features to identify are the duration of the disease, its severity (in terms of peripheral vascular disease, retinopathy and nephropathy), prepregnancy requirements for insulin and current dosage. If possible, identify the quality of glycaemic control around the time of conception. This relies on the patient being a 'complier' who might have planned her pregnancy. Well-motivated diabetics tend to know their glycosylated haemoglobin values, and this is worth asking about.

Ask what measures have been taken during pregnancy to identify retinopathy and nephropathy. Ask directly about when the eyes were last formally examined.

The family history is occasionally relevant in type 1 diabetes, and should be asked about.

The history of the current pregnancy is important. Menstrual upset is commoner in diabetics and the gestation at booking is important.

It is worth including in your history a note of how the insulin requirements have increased. The name of the diabetic physician is also worth knowing, as he or she plays a crucial role in the antenatal care.

EXAMINATION

Your general examination should address problems such as assessing vascular disease (the chances of finding a pregnant diabetic with significant vasculopathy is very small indeed, but nevertheless make a point of commenting on the normality of the capillary return). You must examine the retinas and comment on them. It is likely that you will know considerably more about the diabetic retina than your examiners. Pre-eclampsia is common in diabetics: check the blood pressure carefully.

Abdominal palpation is directed at identifying a macrosomic fetus or polyhydramnios. Alternatively, you may find no abnormality or even evidence of IUGR if the disease is poorly controlled and there is small vessel disease. Measure the abdominal girth and elicit or exclude a fluid thrill.

FACTFILE

1. Fetal anomaly is less common in women attending prepregnancy clinics for diabetics than those who do not attend.
2. HbA levels of more than 12% are associated with increased rates of fetal anomaly, particularly neural tube defect and cardiac disease.

DISCUSSION POINTS

1. The normal physiology of glucose control is beloved of some people and you ought to be familiar with both the pattern of normal renal clearance in pregnancy and the pattern of insulin secretion in pregnancy.
2. The criteria for normality of a glucose tolerance test and how you might perform such a test provide useful starting points for discussion, as does the value of screening the normal population for impaired glucose tolerance in pregnancy.

PREVIOUS FETAL LOSS/ABNORMALITY ★

DEFINITIONS

- **Miscarriage**   The termination of a pregnancy before 24 weeks' gestation that results in the expulsion of a fetus that shows no signs of life.
- **Stillbirth**   The delivery after 24 weeks' gestation of a fetus that shows no sign of life.
- **Early neonatal death**   Death within 1 week of delivery of a live newborn, regardless of the gestational age at delivery.
- **Late neonatal death**   Death between 1 and 4 weeks of a newborn, regardless of the gestational age at delivery.
- **Perinatally related infant death**   Death of an infant between 4 weeks and 1 year of life from a cause that was perinatally related.

PRINCIPAL CAUSES

- Intrauterine growth restriction   ★★★
- Fetal abnormality   ★★
- Prematurity   ★★★
- Infection   ★
- Maternal hypertension   ★★
- Trauma   ★
- Antepartum haemorrhage   ★★★

HISTORY

The history taking should be directed at identifying the cause of the previous loss or the nature of the fetal abnormality. This may require even more sensitivity than you normally use. Identify the measures that have been taken to identify or exclude a recurrence of the problem.

EXAMINATION

Although unlikely in clinical finals, if you do get a case of previous loss then examination is directed at identifying or excluding signs of recurrence.

DISCUSSION POINT

You should be able to describe the relative contributions that, for example, fetal abnormality and infection contribute to perinatal mortality rates. You should know the perinatal mortality rate in the hospitals in which you have undertaken your obstetric attachment.

RHESUS DISEASE ★

DEFINITION

A condition wherein maternal IgG class antibodies cause fetal haemolysis, most commonly because of previous maternal exposure to rhesus D antigen. Other antigens can cause haemolysis, and many of the principles of the management of rhesus disease are common to other antigens.

HISTORY

Previous exposure is required in order for a woman to become isoimmunized. This is commonly from previous pregnancies. Improperly matched blood transfusion is rare. Failure of prophylaxis, either administrative or true therapeutic failure, is becoming the most important cause of rhesus disease in the UK. Determine the likely sensitizing event. Failure to administer anti-D prophylaxis following previous termination of pregnancy should not be forgotten. If the patient has undergone previous abortion or miscarriage she should be aware of whether anti-D was given. If she is not, there may be a number of possible explanations (such as poor memory), but nevertheless this is an important point to make to the examiners.

Check whether the patient is aware of the likely genotype of her partner. Useful questions relate to whether she has been told that the baby will definitely be affected (partner homozygous D) or if there is only a 50% chance (partner heterozygous). If you are lucky, she may also be aware of the titre of antibody or quantitation.

The past obstetric history should be very clearly presented. Specifically, find out how badly affected previous babies were and at what gestations invasive investigations or treatments were begun. Find out what investigations relevant to the diagnosis have been made in the current pregnancy. If, for example, amniocentesis has already been performed, find out at what gestation. Fetal blood sampling may have been performed, either diagnostically or for the purposes of intravascular transfusion. The significance of the gestation at delivery and whether this was iatrogenic is worthy of emphasis, as is the duration of stay for the baby in the neonatal unit and the number of exchange transfusions (if the mother is aware of this).

EXAMINATION

Remember that isoimmunization is a disease of the fetus rather than of the mother, so general examination will usually be unremarkable.

FACTFILE

1. 1% of rhesus negative women become isoimmunized during pregnancy. Antepartum administration of anti-D reduces this frequency to about 0.3%.
2. As rhesus D problems reduce, the incidence of other red cell antigens causing problems is increasing. These are Kell, anti-

C, anti-c and anti-E. Other antigens may also cause haemolysis, but are relatively rare.
3. 500 IU of anti-D covers a fetomaternal haemorrhage of 4 ml.

DISCUSSION POINTS

1. Discussion of the management of non-sensitized rhesus-negative women during pregnancy is as likely as a question on the management of rhesus disease.

2. The indications for and dosage of anti-D may be mentioned in connection with a number of cases. For example, if you present a case of antepartum haemorrhage in a rhesus-negative woman you must mention the need for anti-D.

PAEDIATRICS

HISTORY AND EXAMINATION IN PAEDIATRICS

The clinical examination in paediatrics differs from the others in many respects. The first of these is that you must establish a relationship with a child or infant, as well as with the parents and examiners. Many medical schools have abandoned long cases in paediatrics and replaced them with a series of short cases. This means that you must establish your relationship with the patient quickly, as you will still need to take a history as well as perform competent clinical examination and elicit clinical signs.

You must have practised communicating with children before the exams. Your results will be better if you know basic facts and can demonstrate that you do not have every 5-year-old running away from you, than if you know every obscure paediatric syndrome but every child you see hides under mother's coat until you have gone away!

At this point it is worth pointing out that your demeanour is best directed at the patient. Modern paediatric wards are fairly informal places, and much has been written about how doctors are perceived by children. Your approach to the examiners must always be formal, but you can approach the child, through his or her parents, in an informal fashion.

EQUIPMENT

You will already possess a stethoscope and tendon hammer and perhaps even your own ophthalmoscope. In paediatrics it is more important to possess a tape measure than a tendon hammer. A torch is equally important. In order to impress the examiners it is worth bringing some children's bricks or toys to attract the child's attention and perform developmental assessment if needed. Borrow these if necessary.

HISTORY TAKING

When you take the history a parent will often be available. The important thing here is never to approach the child directly. You must demonstrate to the child that his or her parent is comfortable with you and that you are no kind of threat. With younger children you should avoid starting off by asking direct questions of the child, as this can result in a clam-like attitude on their part. The parent will then only respond to the anxieties provoked in their child, so you have lost their confidence too. This remains a good rule even with older children.

When you take the history this must be from the very beginning, i.e. the history of the pregnancy. Particular attention should be paid to the occurrence of any complications during the pregnancy, the mode of delivery and, crucially, the gestational age at delivery. Admission to a neonatal unit and duration of stay is also important.

A developmental history should be taken and may even be the point of one of the cases. You should know how to do this already, but in essence the milestones of smiling, standing, independent walking and acquisition of hand skills should be documented. Remember always to relate this to gestationally adjusted age and not to age from birth. It follows that you must know the normal age of reaching these milestones.

Nutrition is important and you should identify the quality and quantity of the child's eating pattern. This applies to infant feeding as well the older child, and you should certainly know whether the baby was breastfed or not. In connection with this you must be familiar with the growth charts used in paediatrics. If you are presented with one and do not have a clue about the meanings of centile values and how the charts are used (including correction for gestational age) then you create a very poor impression, as these are fundamental in paediatric practice.

Family history is important in this connection, as parental size may be important. Other aspects of the family history are as important as in any other field, but there are certain clues that should be sought and the behaviour and health of siblings are important. There may be other relatives with related problems. These may be forgotten by parents, and it is worth asking if any relatives had health problems in childhood, attended special schools or had special educational needs.

Social history is of obvious importance, but specific enquiry should be made about whether the parents smoke. This requires tact and caution: you should not alienate the parents, on whom you rely for further information.

In older children ask about school absence and performance.

You should have mastered the other aspects of history taking, but their application in paediatrics requires practice.

EXAMINATION: LONG CASES

Before you begin to examine the patient you must already have established a relationship with both parent – usually the mother – and child. Remember to smile. This is so basic, but very difficult if you yourself are feeling a little strained because of the examination. Once again, practice and familiarity with examining children should help. Ask the mother if you may examine her child. The child must realize that this stranger is not a threat and that mother agrees to the examination. Once you have established this, speak to the child. This is by no means easy, and it is important to take note of the child's response. A child who is very shy may be so naturally, or be frightened by you, or hospitals, or by adults generally. This may be a clue to significant underlying problems and may be worthy of later comment. Similarly an overly affectionate child, looking for love and attention, may also be expressing underlying problems.

Be nice to the patient. This little person is probably a lot more anxious than you are and really does not care about your worries. If you are kind to the child in the finals you will keep your examiners happy even if you do not know the minutiae. Always remember this.

Finally, if you are seeing more than one patient in the exam, for example between short cases, you must remember to wash your hands between patients unless you are instructed to the contrary.

GENERAL PHYSICAL EXAMINATION

There are a few general points that you should have reached before you examine the child formally. While you have been taking the history you should already have formed an impression of whether the child has any dysmorphic features. These may be obvious, as in Down syndrome. Less immediately obvious, at least at the outset, will be features such as whether the head is proportionate in size to the trunk.

You will know the child's age, chronological and gestationally adjusted, and you should know if he or she is small for his or her age. This depends on your knowledge of the normal range of size for children of a given age. Failure to identify a significant discrepancy in size for age is a sure indication to the examiners that your presence on the wards has been less than colossal.

Take note of the child's response to you and the other adults. Is he or she withdrawn or suspicious? When you begin the examination, always ask for the mother's help to undress the child – not to restrain but to encourage the child (if possible). It is important to mention that there is no absolutely correct way to perform a physical examination in paediatrics. Much of the examination might be made in an opportunistic fashion. A systematic approach or a 'top to tail' approach may be attempted, but success with either depends on a huge number of variables. Your capacity to adapt will again indicate to the examiners that you are not new to the difficulties of examining children.

It is fair to say that you will rarely be asked to perform a detailed general examination. It is more likely that you will be instructed to listen to or examine the child's chest. You should still take note of all the other clues mentioned above.

For clarity of layout the examination style presented below will follow a systematic approach.

Cardiovascular system

Look for the obvious things, such as clubbing and cyanosis. Distinguish peripheral from central cyanosis. Tachypnoea may also be a more obvious sign of cardiac disease than in the adult.

Check both arm pulses: one absent radial pulse is distinctly possible in a child who has undergone surgery for Fallot's tetralogy. Similarly, feel the femoral pulses: absent or poor-quality femoral pulses raise the possibility of coarctation of the aorta. Generally you will not be asked to check the BP, but you should know generalities about the automatic BP monitors that are used so much in paediatrics.

Palpate the chest before auscultation. Cardiac thrills are often pronounced in children and the site of the apex beat must be identified. Do not get too excited about the characteristics of any murmurs. You should know the basics, so do try to identify systolic or diastolic murmurs but do not panic if it all sounds very complicated. Paediatric cardiologists use echocardiography, so they obviously find some of the sounds confusing! You should, however, know how to grade a murmur. Remember that you may be asked to examine a normal child. Flow murmurs are common!

Remember to look for scars on the chest. A sternal thoracotomy usually means surgery for either a VSD or complex heart disease. A lateral thoracotomy usually indicates a persistent ductus arteriosus, a shunt for Fallot's tetralogy or surgery for aortic coarctation.

Respiratory system

Make a point of counting the respiratory rate and identifying intercostal and sternal recession. As in cardiac disease, you should identify clubbing if present. It is unlikely that you will see a case such as severe asthma, but do remember that the asthmatic child without a wheeze who cannot talk is probably very much sicker than a wheezy talker.

In children younger than 1 year old percussion of the chest is not very helpful and may frighten the child. In older children it may be helpful. Auscultation of the chest is usually helpful, but possibly less so in infants. You should be aware of how to measure peak expiratory flow using Wright's peak flow meter. You should also be familiar with the various types of inhalers, spacer devices and nebulizers.

The observation that a child is receiving oxygen by nasal cannula is worth comment, and if in addition the child has a hyperinflated chest, is less than a year old and is small, should ring an alarm bell that says this child is a survivor of prematurity with bronchopulmonary dysplasia.

Abdominal examination

Treat the paediatric abdomen with gentleness. Cold hands and too firm an initial touch will result in a disgruntled and uncooperative patient. Do not hurry this bit of the examination. Talk to the child gently and quietly while you examine. This also ensures that you are looking at the child's face rather than the abdomen as you palpate, and this is important. The initial palpation must be very superficial in every sense, as the spleen in particular can be readily felt if enlarged. Roll the child on to his or her right side to increase further the prospects of identifying a splenic problem. Remember to feel for the lower border of the liver and, if appropriate, percuss for the upper limit.

Comment on scars, looking for hernias or access for transplants.

Once confidence is established (both yours and the child's) you can palpate more deeply. Ticklish children are a problem, but often the examiners will recognize this and, if you are lucky, direct you to something else. If you think there is ascites then involve the examiner or parent in helping you elicit a fluid thrill.

Never ever forget to examine the hernial orifices. This might be the point of the whole exam, so do not forget.

You should also make an attempt to examine the genitalia (but only in the presence of the parents or examiners). If the child is dressed you should say, for example, that you would like to remove the nappy. This in itself might be all the examiners want to hear and they may not even ask you to continue, but do mention it. If you are asked to examine for undescended testes it is important to get the child to sit and to attempt to 'milk' the testes down the inguinal canal.

Skin

Any rashes in paediatric exams are likely to be eczema, psoriasis or possibly Henoch–Schönlein purpura. The infectious causes are very unlikely, as most paediatricians do not want rip-roaring chickenpox going through their wards. The one 'infectious' condition you might see is scabies, so remember to examine the feet and hands carefully.

You might occasionally see a case of Stevens–Johnson syndrome, so try to obtain a drug history if possible.

Café au lait spots of neurofibromatosis may also be seen.

Limbs

You may be asked to examine the limbs. This is difficult, as if you have no history you may be uncertain whether the problem is an orthopaedic one, such as Perthes' disease, neurological, such as spina bifida (always examine the back), or an arthritis.

If the patient is old enough then try to assess the gait. You should know how to measure the limbs and check both for asymmetry in size, but also for muscle wasting.

Isolated arthritis is a possible but unlikely case. Check for joint effusions. You must distinguish between acute and chronic arthritis.

Central nervous system

This is so interwoven with developmental assessment and examination of the limbs that you may already have reached a neurological diagnosis. First, take note of the size of the head and determine whether it is in proportion to the body. Measure the occipitofrontal circumference. Look for a ventriculoperitoneal shunt.

Neurological conditions in paediatrics can be complex, but the examiners do not want or expect you to identify obscure syndromes. Make all the relevant observations, but if you are unable to identify a common aetiology then do not panic.

Assess tone. You should recognize increased or decreased tone.

Assess power. Be sensible: if the child can walk without any problem then it is unlikely that there is any significant loss of power in the lower limbs.

In younger children you must be able to demonstrate primitive reflexes and know when they disappear. In older children clonus and mature reflexes should be elicited. The plantar reflex requires some sensitivity in use in children.

Examination of the eyes is important. Look particularly for squint and know the cover test. Using an ophthalmoscope can be challenging in paediatrics. The examiners will not expect you to identify any obscure problems, but you should appear confident in the use of this instrument. Once again, practice and familiarity are the keys. Do not battle with the child to examine the fundi. If you must, then solicit the aid of the parents, or even the examiners. Do not hold the child's head still yourself. This may be frightening for the child and indeed the parents. Be flexible: you may only have the opportunity for a quick glimpse, but make use of it.

Cataracts would be an unlikely finding but you should look for these as well as any obvious nystagmus. Be able to recognize a normal red reflex.

If you are asked to examine the eyes then the odds are high that you will be asked about the nerves and muscles involved in eye movement. If you have not read this recently and do not remember them, then do so now! Always comment on whether squints are paralytic or not and check visual acuity in case of amblyopia.

Developmental assessment

It is very likely that you will be asked to perform a developmental assessment on any child. It is important to be aware that this does not necessarily mean that there is anything actually wrong with the child. Healthy children may take part in the examination.

Usually in such a case the patient will be 3 years old or younger. You will be asked to assess developmental age. This might provoke a question such as 'Why is this 3-year-old child performing at a 15-month level?'

Try to be logical in your assessment: if the child is sitting down and playing with a toy then it is time-wasting to talk about testing for appropriate smiling responses or head control and primitive reflexes.

If the child is not playing then use any (safe) articles lying around. If you have seen the child demonstrate pincer grasp during play then do not repeat this. You might not get the child to perform for you! Obviously a lot of developmental assessment is done fortuitously while watching the child.

Make note of the major areas: fine and gross motor skills can be assessed at play; vision and hand coordination likewise. Hearing and language may have to be more formally tested, so have a system for doing this. Social development can be difficult to determine in the context of a hospital, and also of a clinical examination such as the finals. A child who is obviously mixing with other children on the ward is easier to assess in this regard than the shy or withdrawn child, and this may be worth commenting upon to the examiners.

THE CASES

In contrast with the other final examination disciplines it is not as readily possible to present definitions or presentation of cases by symptomatology. A number of different conditions may present with a common range of symptoms. A history may be impossible to obtain and may appear to conflict with other clinical evidence. For example, you may be presented with a child who looks wasted and is failing to thrive but whose mother says the child is well and eats voraciously. This of course should raise clinical suspicions but can be difficult for you to deal with during a clinical examination.

It is worth commenting that it would be quite unusual, though not impossible, to be presented with a newborn baby. Similarly, think of how likely certain conditions are to come up if you are sitting the exam during the spring or summer months: although you should know all about bronchiolitis, the chance of getting a case between May and July is negligible.

CARDIAC DISEASE ★★★★★

The two principal types of cardiac disease are *cyanotic* and *acyanotic*. Cyanotic disease is most commonly Fallot's tetralogy (★★★★) or some complex heart disease (★★★★). It is unlikely that you would see one of the other causes of cyanosis and you would not be expected to make a diagnosis.

Symptoms as reported by parents are very important. Has the cyanosis been present from birth? Have there been feeding problems and colour changes with feeding? Parents may think that previous surgery is so obvious that they do not mention it to you, so be very clear about this aspect of the history.

On examination you want to identify whether there is cyanosis. If there is, then carefully distinguish between central and peripheral cyanosis. This is important both clinically and in the exam. Feel both radial arteries, especially if there is a history of previous surgery. Feel the femoral pulses. If you have to remove or move underwear to do this then enlist the help of the parents.

Palpate the chest for thrills and for the apex beat, as these can be more pronounced in children than in adults. Another difference to be aware of is that children in cardiac failure do not usually have peripheral oedema but may well have more obvious liver enlargement.

Look for 'syndromes': trisomy 21 and trisomy 18 are both associated with complex cardiac lesions. Turner's syndrome is associated with aortic coarctation and aortic stenosis.

FACTFILE

1. The commonest causes of acyanotic heart disease are ventricular septal defect, pulmonary stenosis, atrial septal defect, patent ductus arteriosus, aortic stenosis and coarctation of the aorta.
2. Around 12% of children with congenital cardiac problems have more than one heart defect.
3. Rheumatic heart disease is now rare in western practice, but may be seen in immigrant communities.

Discussion points

1. The investigations that might be undertaken in paediatric cardiology include echocardiography and Doppler examination of the vessels and flow across the valves. You need not know about these in detail, but should be familiar with the principles.
2. It is important to know the principles behind antibiotic prophylaxis for children with cardiac disease. Similarly, the management of subacute bacterial endocarditis should be familiar to you.
3. Newer, minimally invasive techniques of treating obstructive cardiac disease are becoming established and you may be asked about these.
4. Many heart murmurs are innocent in children, and you might be asked what advice you would give the parents of a child with such a finding.

DEVELOPMENTAL DELAY ★★★★

A child who fails to reach the milestones in the major developmental areas within the normal range is said to exhibit developmental delay. The causes are numerous but, as previously discussed, the birth and family history are particularly important. Social interaction is important, and developmental delay may result from poor stimulation and can result in a child who is clearly failing to thrive.

It is worth repeating that you must know the major milestones. If you think that unintelligible babble is appropriate for a 26-month-old child then you have a problem, as the examiners will think that you and the child share some characteristics, i.e. your contribution may be unintelligible babble to them!

If possible, your general examination should be linked with the developmental assessment, and this highlights that a lot of paediatric examination technique is opportunistic.

FACTFILE

1. Many causes of developmental delay can be screened for, and congenital hypothyroidism and phenylketonuria are good examples. About one in 3500 children is affected by hypothyroidism, and although some may already be damaged in utero, early treatment is effective in preventing deterioration in these cases and in preventing adverse effects in the remainder.

2. Phenylketonuria was one of the first metabolic disorders to be treated to prevent significant handicap. Approximately one baby in 14 000 will be identified in screening programmes.

3. Metabolic disorders are not particularly common but may be referred to tertiary centres, and these are often where the exam is held. Be warned! Do not waste time trying to remember details about them.

Discussion points

1. Environmental effects on childhood development are currently being emphasized in both the lay and the medical literature. You may be asked to comment on which aspect

of the environment is the greatest contributor to developmental delay.

2. What single aspect of medical care may improve the outcome in developmental delay?

3. The interaction of the child with other members of the family and family stress may promote problems with development. How might these be alleviated?

4. It is very important to be aware of and able to discuss, at least superficially, the many different disciplines involved in the care of the handicapped child. Neurologists, ophthalmologists, psychologists and many therapists as well as paediatricians, will contribute to the care of these children.

NEUROLOGICAL DISORDERS ★★★★★

The cases that might present under this heading are variable. The most likely are cerebral palsy (motor disorder) ★★★★★ or spina bifida ★★. You may be presented with an epileptic child, although this is unlikely. In practical terms it may be easier for exam organizers to find a child admitted with febrile convulsions.

The history should be relatively straightforward. Although the vast majority of cerebral palsy is unrelated to intrapartum events, you must obtain a comprehensive birth history. A history of prematurity and prolonged early hospitalization is very important. You should know the different types of cerebral palsy, e.g. hemiplegic, diplegic and so on.

The family and social history is important in these cases. How is the family as a whole coping? The educational needs of the child should be discussed and any plans the parents have formed outlined.

Your examination should determine the degree of

handicap. If you are asked to examine a child whose head looks disproportionately large, then do remember that hydrocephalus still occurs. When you examine such a child make sure to check the site of the shunt. It is also worth measuring the parental head size if possible.

Assess the degree of the child's mobility.

THE SCRAWNY/SMALL CHILD ★★★★

You may be presented with a child who is failing to thrive. In an OSCE station you may be presented with a photograph of a child who is obviously failing to thrive or a growth chart. In a long case your history should identify any obvious genetic points and the child's initial development. The principal points during examination relate to whether the child is appropriately nourished and proportionately small. This kind of child may be a constitutionally small child, whereas the findings of muscle wasting with a distended abdomen suggest an organic problem.

In a little girl remember the possibility of Turner's syndrome. Endocrine problems such as growth hormone deficiency and hypothyroidism are not common, but the examiners will be happy to discuss these treatable problems.

Social history is very important in these children, as failure to thrive is not infrequently associated with neglect.

It is essential to correlate your findings to growth charts. If you are presented with a small child and have not used the appropriate growth charts or suggested their use you will fail (or deserve to). Disproportionate smallness may be due to achondroplasia, so assess long bone length.

FACTFILE

1. In a Newcastle community study of 98 children below the third centile for height there were six chromosomal problems, one case each of cystic fibrosis, chronic renal failure, cyanotic congenital cardiac disease, growth hormone deficiency and Hurler's syndrome, and four defined as mental handicap.

2. Coeliac disease is a rare but recognized cause of small stature. The incidence appears to be reducing, possibly owing to a reduction in childhood exposure to dietary allergens.

3. Congenital hypothyroidism should be excluded by the introduction of neonatal screening, so the majority of hypothyroid cases are juveniles.

4. Birth length is doubled at age 4 and trebled by the age of 13.

Discussion points

1. You will be expected to be familiar with growth charts and how they are used.

2. The role of the environment in childhood growth and development is important and may well be discussed.

3. The investigation of the small child is a reasonable topic, but because it can appear all-embracing it is important to have a clear idea of what is involved and not to jump to invasive tests too early.

THE BREATHLESS CHILD ★★★

Breathlessness may be a factor in many different paediatric problems. These can be infectious, such as bronchiolitis (★★★, but remember this is seasonal), environmental/genetic, such as asthma (★★★★★), or genetic, such as cystic fibrosis (★★★★) or as a consequence of prematurity i.e. chronic lung disease. Heart defects may also present with breathlessness.

The history should be directed towards identifying the most likely underlying problem, such as a genetic or family history, as in cystic fibrosis, or a family history of atopy. Social history is important. Establish whether the parents smoke. This can be difficult because, as previously mentioned, you must try not to alienate the parents.

Drug history is important. If the child uses inhalers try to identify how suitable this is for a child of his or her age. Some children are given standard inhalers when patient-triggered or spacer devices would be much more effective. Find out if prophylactic treatment is being given and get some idea of compliance (on the part of either the child or the parent).

On examination assess growth. All children with severe underlying disease are likely to have some impairment of growth. This is especially likely in children with cystic fibrosis. Look for other signs: clubbing may be seen.

A good clue to chronic lung disease is oxygen dependency.

FACTFILE

1. 13% of children with cystic fibrosis will not present until they are 5 years old or older.

2. Half of all children with cystic fibrosis will present before 6 months of age. Most will present with respiratory illness or failure to thrive because of malabsorption.

3. Acute bronchiolitis is usually a winter disease, and implicated viruses include parainfluenza, rhino- and adenoviruses, although the respiratory syncytial virus is the best-remembered one.

4. The incidence of asthma is increasing dramatically. Air pollution is not the only cause, but environmental factors do appear to be very significant, particularly parental smoking.

Discussion points

1. You may be asked about the different types of inhaler that might be used in children.

2. The difference between the treatment of acute asthma and ongoing management with maintenance is sometimes blurred in difficult cases, but you should be able to distinguish what you mean by these terms.

3. Peak flow meters are important in assessing the older child. Know how to use one. A useful test for examiners is to ask candidates how they would instruct a child to use a peak flow meter. If you have not 'been around' this can be tricky.

DYSMORPHISM ★★★★

In large teaching hospitals in particular, medical students may leave paediatrics with the impression that the specialty is preoccupied with syndromes. This is not true, but there are a number of syndromes with which you should be familiar. These are Down syndrome (★★★★★), Edward syndrome (★), Turner's syndrome (★★★) and Klinefelter's syndrome (★). There are other syndromes that you may see during teaching. A small hint is that, if they are rare and chronic with prolonged hospitalization, you may see the same child in the exam!

In your history and examination you should aim to identify the specific abnormalities the child has. Even if you have the greatest mental blank and cannot remember the common name of trisomy 21, you should comment on developmental delay, the presence of a heart defect, floppiness and characteristic facies. Put another way, the examiners will not care too much if you cannot remember Treacher–Collins syndrome if you can summarize the clinical features the patient presents.

Your history should identify what medical, social, family and educational problems the family is experiencing in bringing up their child. If you have time it is worth identifying the effects, if any, on siblings.

LUMPS AND BUMPS ★★★★

Many medical schools also include paediatric surgical cases in the finals. You may be asked to examine the abdomen. Make a point of identifying organomegaly (★★★★★). Hernial (★★★★★) orifices must be checked. Umbilical hernias (★★★★) are very common, though, and you should know that they only very rarely require surgery. Consequently, if presented with such a case and you have the opportunity, try to find out whether there is any other reason for the child being in hospital. This may get you some Brownie points.

Groin hernias in boys are commonly inguinal, but in girls they may also be femoral.

You should recognize hydroceles (★★★★★) and also be aware of the difference between maldescent and undescent of the testes. Once again, the need for the cooperation of parents in this aspect of the examination cannot be overemphasized.

SKIN PROBLEMS ★★★

You may be asked to examine a rash or skin lesion, and your description should use the standard dermatological terms of papular, macular, erythematous, etc. At the end of your description you should be able to reach some kind of diagnosis, the commonest of which are ammoniacal dermatitis (★★★★), atopic eczema (★★★★★) and the various types of naevus (★★★★★). Psoriasis (★★) may also be seen.

Infectious causes may also be seen, so look between the fingers and on the feet for scabies and warts. Head lice have not been eradicated so do look, just in case.

Psoriasis may also be present on the scalp, and is important to comment upon if so.

History should identify the aetiological factors. Atopy is important and a specific family history should be sought. Similarly, any obvious allergens should be identified if possible.

PAINFUL JOINT(S) ★★

Painful swollen joints are more likely to be rheumatic than septic in origin. Rheumatoid arthritis, juvenile and pauciarticular are the most common types.

Post-infectious painful joints occur following rheumatic fever, but this is now rare. Allergic phenomena such as Henoch–Schönlein purpura may present with joint pain. Haemorrhagic disorders such as haemophilia can cause long-standing joint disruption, as can leukaemia. Your history taking should be directed at identifying the likely cause, e.g. Was there a history of recent viral illness? Is the child known to be haemophiliac? Have there been previous admissions for treatment (suggesting an ongoing, possibly rheumatic origin)?

Your examination should illustrate your concern not to hurt the child, but you should elicit the clinical signs. Remember to check for effusions at the knees and point out associated muscle wasting.

Other causes of painful joints or limp may be presented. Transient synovitis follows a viral infection but can be difficult to distinguish from Perthes' disease when the hip is involved.

FACTFILE

1. About 6% of children thought to have transient synovitis develop Perthes' disease.

2. The sequelae of missing the diagnosis of congenital hip dislo-cation are severe. Babies born by breech delivery are at increased risk.
3. Scoliosis of the spine is a curvature of the spine in the coronal plane; the majority are idiopathic and occur in females.
4. Accidents are the single greatest contributor to mortality rates in children between the ages of 3 and 14.

Discussion points

1. You must know the available tests for screening for hip dislocation. Ultrasound examination of the hip has become popular, but its role is as yet uncertain, although large trials are addressing this.
2. Club foot occurs in around one per 1000 births. Treatment is difficult and prolonged. You should know the different types and the procedures available for management.
3. *Staphylococcus pyogenes* is the commonest organism in osteomyelitis. The diagnostic indicators are important and you should know them. Do not mention X-rays as being initially valuable: only students who have not been around think they are. Radiological changes in acute osteomyelitis are not obvious within the first 10 days of presentation.
4. Know the difference between osteogenesis imperfecta and osteochondritis. For some reason some students confuse these very different conditions.
5. Painful joints may also follow trauma. This can lead on to discussion of topics such as accident prevention in paediatrics. This is an area of increasing importance. Similarly, the trauma may not have been that much of an accident and you may end up discussing non-accidental injury and at-risk registers.

AND FINALLY

Repetition of this does no harm: smile at the child and be nice!

PSYCHIATRY

HISTORY AND EXAMINATION IN PSYCHIATRY

The General Medical Council's guidance on medical education, as published in 1997, highlighted the frequency with which medical students in many different fields see patients with psychiatric disorders. This encouraged a reassessment of the place of psychiatry within the undergraduate curriculum and most UK university medical courses now incorporate psychiatry into their undergraduate teaching on a par with other major specialities. Psychiatry is, therefore, not only a specialty in its own right, but is now generally recognized as an important constituent part of medical training and hence a subject for inclusion in clinical finals.

EXAMINATION FORMAT

OSCEs and objectively assessed long cases have an increasingly important role to play in the assessment of medical students' clinical skills. Many medical students attending UK universities will sit at least one psychiatry OSCE as part of their finals and may well meet a psychiatric long case.

This chapter will first provide a brief introduction to the discipline of psychiatry to help students prepare for finals. This section will explain views on current approaches in psychiatry, specify some of the more important ways in which psychiatry differs from other medical subjects, highlight factors that relate specifically to psychiatry and outline some of the key skills and knowledge that students should have mastered during their psychiatry placements. A succinct, general guide to the two main assessment tools used by psychiatrists, that is the Core Psychiatric Assessment and the Mental State Examination, as well as a brief guide to developing a care management plan will be given. This will be followed by a brief synopsis of the key disorders, listed alphabetically under broad headings, such as affective disorders. Each topic area adheres to the general format of the rest of the text, incorporating specific information on definitions, history taking, assessment, a 'factfile' and discussion points for each individual case.

Diagnosis may also be complicated by comorbidity, mental or physical, in a substantial proportion of psychiatric illnesses. There is no intention to produce a fully comprehensive list of every psychiatric diagnosis that could appear in a clinical examination in one chapter. As with other contributions to this book, this text is intended as a guide to consolidate past independent study on the part of the student and to facilitate a broader programme of revision. It does, nevertheless, attempt to cover the major subject areas in psychiatry that are most likely to appear.

For this section summary points and brief definitions have been used wherever possible in place of substantial blocks of text. The selection of cases for this chapter has been based upon what students actually covered while on their psychiatry rotations, the class curricula for psychiatry blocks and examples from past examinations, and finally, on the opinions of a number of consultant psychiatrists who teach medical students and set exams. For this section all conditions should be considered as possible OSCEs or long case examinations.

THE BIOPSYCHOSOCIAL MODEL OF PSYCHIATRY

Despite being widely regarded as a necessary part of general medical training, psychiatry is distinct from most other medical specialties in several ways. Not least among these differences is the wide acceptance of the 'biopsychosocial model' of aetiology. This perspective essentially argues that biological, psychological and social factors all have a role to play in the pathogenesis, and therefore the treatment, of psychiatric conditions and thus allows for a holistic approach to treatment. This differs from the prevailing school of thought earlier in the twentieth century which favoured the so-called 'biological model'. The central tenet of the biological model is that effective treatments are those that change the physical state of the body in such a way as to correct the physical cause of the illness. This model has been criticized as excluding, or at best marginalizing, the importance of psychological and social factors. The biopsychosocial model has now become accepted among psychiatrists and is familiar to most mental health workers.

There are, however, three main criticisms of the biopsychosocial model. The first arises largely as a result of developments in areas such as brain imaging and molecular genetics, which have emphasized the importance of genetic and other biological factors. The second criticism relates to the application of the biopsychosocial model; the perceived use of the model to justify the pragmatic application of numerous different treatments by a variety of mental health workers. The final criticism made of the model is that it is simply an extension of the biological model, with the incorporation of social and psychological factors. Regardless of these criticisms, the model remains the dominant paradigm upon which psychiatry is practiced in the early twenty-first century. By applying this model, students have a useful framework for considering questions put to them on aetiology and treatment. By addressing

PSYCHIATRY

such issues under the subheadings of 'biological, psychological and social' factors, the student will have more chance of impressing examiners.

ASSESSING PSYCHIATRIC PATIENTS IN CLINICAL FINALS

Psychiatry aims to achieve an understanding of psychiatric conditions and their treatment. Nevertheless, there are important differences from other specialties due to the nature of psychiatric illness, the way in which diagnosis is determined and the treatments offered to patients. In psychiatry there is much greater emphasis upon verbal assessment skills, such as history taking. This is because diagnosis and prognosis rely heavily upon information gathered at interview with the patient and significant others. Reliable individuals who can provide information about the context, nature and extent of the illness may include a relative or carer, the patient's family doctor or other health professionals. Due to practical difficulties, it is unlikely that students would be expected to elicit such a so-called 'collateral history' in a clinical examination setting. Nonetheless, examiners will expect students to recognize the importance of this source of information and to state that, given the opportunity, they would want to talk to such individuals.

The ability to gain the confidence of patients is also imperative to a successful verbal assessment. This skill is even more important in psychiatry than in other fields of medicine because of the importance of the information that is being elicited and often the absence of other sources of information, such as laboratory investigations. The examiners will assess the candidate's ability to attain the relevant information, understand the causes and context of the disorder and form a therapeutic relationship with the patient.

As well as taking a comprehensive psychiatric history and mental state examination, a general medical examination is also essential. In psychiatry, time constraints usually mean that the focus will be upon the psychiatric assessment. Candidates will also need to show an appreciation of physical health problems, particularly if related to psychiatric disorder. This could include evidence of self-harm, alcohol or drug misuse, or self-neglect, and an appreciation of any relevant physical illness.

'STANDARDIZED' PATIENTS

There is, of course, no such thing as a 'standardized' patient; however, it is becoming increasingly common to use professional actors as a way of standardizing clinical tests. This practice reduces the need for 'real' patients to take part in clinical examinations. Remember that, during clinical finals, while a candidate will see each patient only once, each patient could see several students, each of whom attempts to assess their mental or physical state, or both. Clinical finals can be an exhausting and distressing experience for patients as well as for students! The use of standardized patients also has many practical benefits. As well as allowing examiners to plan the examination in advance and alleviating the stress on patients, using actors reduces many of the potential variables associated with clinical exams. This helps ensure that each student is faced with a similar scenario, across and within sites.

At this point it is useful to think about some of the practicalities associated with using actors in psychiatry OSCEs. A simulated patient is able to simulate, for example, depressive disorder: they could be unshaven, have slowed speech and avoid eye contact. It is highly unlikely, however, that they would present signs of self-harm or weight loss. Simulated patients will usually follow a 'script'. The advantage to candidates is that simulated patients are far less likely to mislead or provide irrelevant information. Nevertheless, the actor will expect the student to ask the appropriate questions to elicit key information. It also means, however, that if you are familiar with the standard assessment tools used in psychiatry and have an empathic approach, you should have less difficulty in ascertaining the information you require.

PSYCHIATRIC ASSESSMENT

It is imperative that all medical students are proficient in performing the core psychiatric assessment and mental state examination, and are able to develop a care management plan. This has been kept brief as students should already be familiar with both tools from their psychiatry placements. Remember that in clinical examinations there will usually be inadequate time to undertake a comprehensive psychiatric assessment interview. This is particularly true in OSCEs but may also apply in longer case examinations as well. Furthermore, in an OSCE students are normally given a brief outline that includes an indication of diagnosis that allows them to focus on particular areas of assessment. Students will be expected to be familiar with interview techniques and to be able to use the relevant parts of them in a 'problem-focused' manner, to elicit the required information. This includes not only specific questions relating to the presenting problem but also enquiries about any past psychiatric history, any recent life events, and the family and social history.

Principles of psychiatric assessment

There are three key points that students should bear in mind when embarking upon any psychiatric interview: remember to introduce yourself to the patient at the start of the interview; explain who you are and why you want to talk to them; conclude the interview by thanking the patient and explaining what will happen next.

Try to put the patient at ease as quickly as possible and to be empathic. This will help you elicit more relevant information from the patient. It is imperative that you bear cultural, social and religious differences in mind when making a psychiatric assessment. Some attitudes and behaviours that seem inappropriate may well be entirely normal within the patient's sociocultural or religious background.

If appropriate, you should draw upon alternative sources of information. For example, if a patient gives a history of psychiatric disorder or states that they take particular medication, you should emphasize to the examiner that you would seek corroborating evidence from the patient's family doctor before producing a definitive care plan.

Core psychiatric assessment

Taking a comprehensive history from the patient should help you determine the differential diagnosis.

The presenting complaint

- What were the main problems for the patient when he or she initially presented?
- What is the specific reason for the current presentation?
- When did the problems begin?
- When were they first noticed?
- What helped or made the complaints worse?
- Had the patient experienced any particular life events before or after the condition developed?

It is also quite acceptable for the student to ask patients what the medical staff have told them is wrong with them.

Family history

Does the patient have any first-degree, or other, relatives with psychiatric problems? Producing a brief 'family tree' may well be helpful.

Premorbid personality assessment

It is often advantageous to carry out an assessment of the premorbid personality and consider how this may have affected the patient's presentation during the illness.

Social history

It is essential to ascertain information about the patient's accommodation, financial circumstances, carers, and activities inside and/or outside the home.

Past medical history and past psychiatric history

- Is there evidence of any past or current physical conditions? Consider how these may affect the presenting complaint.
- Has the patient ever presented with psychiatric or psychological difficulties in the past? Were there behavioural problems in childhood?

Medication history

- Is the patient currently taking any medication, either routinely or on a discretionary basis?
- Has the patient ever taken medication for psychiatric complaints? If yes, what was this for and did it help?

Mental state examination

This should provide a snapshot of the patient's behavioural and psychological functioning. Remember to describe the signs and symptoms that you elicit, and avoid labelling as 'normal' or 'abnormal'. It is essential that the MSE is considered under the following headings, and in the order shown below.

Appearance and general behaviour

Describe the dress, physical appearance and behaviour of the patient, commenting on self-care, facial expressions, and how easy it is to establish rapport with the patient.

It will also be useful to note whether the patient seems agitated, distracted, restless, tense, hostile, disinhibited, frightened or preoccupied.

Take note of any motor abnormalities and whether the patient appears disorientated.

Speech (form)

Does that patient talk excessively or only a little? Is the speech pressured? Does he or she speak spontaneously? Is the speech loud or quiet? Is the patient coherent or difficult to follow? Does he or she use strange words or associations? Note any verbatim samples of talk that demonstrate examples of flight of ideas, neologisms, perseveration, etc.

Mood (affect)

- How does the patient respond to direct questions regarding his or her mood or spirits?
- Are there any indications of depression or mania (may also be reflected in appearance or behaviour)?
- Is the patient's mood appropriate throughout the interview? Is a normal range of emotional responses exhibited?

Thought content

Check for evidence of:

- morbid thoughts
- abnormal thoughts (e.g. delusions)
- phobias
- obsessional ruminations
- thoughts of harm to self or others.

Abnormal beliefs/interpretations

Specify the content, mode of onset, degree of fixity. Consider three types:

- in relation to the environment, e.g. ideas of reference, misinterpretations or delusions, paranoid beliefs
- in relation to the body, e.g. ideas/delusions of bodily change
- in relation to self, e.g. delusions of passivity, of influence, of thought broadcasting or insertion.

Abnormal perceptions (hallucinations, illusions)

- **Environmental**: hallucinations or illusions may be auditory, visual, olfactory, tactile; feelings of déjà-vu or derealization
- **Body**: altered bodily sensations, somatic hallucinations
- **Self**: depersonalization

Cognitive state

Assess:

- orientation (time, place, person)
- attention and concentration (e.g. serial 7s)

- memory (assess patient's account of recent, past events and ability to recall new information) (It may be helpful to undertake an MMSE).
- intelligence (gauge from history, education, occupation).

Patient's appraisal

It can be useful to explore the patient's perception of the illness. This gives an indication of 'insight'.

DIFFERENTIAL DIAGNOSIS

This should relate to the patient seen, and contain 3–4 possible diagnoses. Students will often be asked for their preferred diagnosis.

Care management plan

In clinical finals students are often asked for their management plan detailing how best to treat the patient they have just assessed. In OSCEs this will usually take the form of a few short questions but in a long case you may well be asked to develop a more comprehensive CMP. There are some key headings that you should consider:

- *Setting* Does this patient need to be admitted? Is he or she appropriate for admission under the Mental Health Act (e.g. patients who pose a risk to themselves, their health, or others)? Admission is sometimes necessary when no suitable alternatives exist.
- *Patient's views* If possible, it is very important to obtain the agreement of patients for their CMP and the patient's views and expectations should be taken into account.
- *Further investigations* What further investigations will be necessary (including case note review and collateral history)?
- *Other professionals* Do you think that the patient would benefit from the involvement of other mental health profes-

sionals, such as a community psychiatric nurse or clinical psychologist? You should be familiar with the roles of the other professionals involved in mental health care.

- *Medication* If you think that medication should be prescribed you should be able to give an example of appropriate medication and dosage, and demonstrate that you are aware of how it acts and the potential side-effects.
- *Comorbidity* Remember to include treatment for any coexisting physical illness in your care plan.

You should have a general awareness of particular diagnostic systems, such as ICD-10, or rating scales, such as the Beck Depression Inventory (BDI) and the Hamilton Rating Scale for Depression or the MMSE for assessing cognition. It is imperative that you are familiar with the terms of the appropriate Mental Health Act and any recent amendments. There is a strong chance that you will be asked whether or not you think a patient should be admitted to hospital and, if so, why. You may further be asked how you would go about admitting this patient, if necessary, under the relevant clause of the Mental Health Act.

Finally, try to avoid using 'labels' with little or no diagnostic value and which can often be misleading or pejorative; for example, talk about 'schizophrenia' not 'schizophrenics'.

Having described the more general information pertinent to psychiatry we shall now describe specific areas of knowledge necessary to pass a clinical examination in psychiatry. Within this section more detailed factual knowledge and specific examples of the questions that should be asked when dealing with particular diagnoses will be given. This information should be incorporated within the framework of the core assessment and MSE. The following notes are not a comprehensive guide to psychiatric diagnoses or a definitive guide to individual examination scenarios. Each section does, however, contain enough relevant information to complement the existing psychiatric knowledge that the student should have acquired, to aid revision and to help negotiate the clinical examination. Good luck!

THE CASES

AFFECTIVE DISORDERS ★★★★★

This term describes a disorder whose main feature is an abnormality of mood, either depression or elation. Affective disorders may or may not be precipitated by traumatic life events. There is also evidence to suggest a genetic component in at least some affective disorders. In severe cases, psychotic symptoms may be present, e.g. delusions of worthlessness.

KEY CLINICAL FEATURES

Depression
- Low mood
- Inability to enjoy normally events or activities
- Feelings of guilt or worthlessness
- Lethargy or agitation, or both
- Negative thoughts
- Pessimism
- Appetite disturbance
- Loss of libido
- Poor concentration, memory or ability to make decisions
- Sleep disruption
- Diurnal variation in mood
- Mood-congruent/mood-incongruent delusions

Mania/Hypomania
- Elated mood
- Feelings of inappropriate happiness

- Distractability
- Disinhibition
- Irritability
- Overactivity
- Self-important ideas (grandiosity)

BIPOLAR AFFECTIVE DISORDER (OR MANIC DEPRESSION) ★★★★★

Some people experience cyclical mood patterns with 'depressive' episodes interspaced with periods of normal mood or elation. Elevations in mood can take the form of mania or, if less severe, hypomania.

Definitions

- **Hypomania** This is characterized by a persistent mild elevation of mood for at least several days. A daily routine is more or less maintained but there may be evidence of increased activity, such as staying up all night to do work; there may be an infectious quality to the sufferer, with increased sociability, talkativeness, overfamiliarity, increased sexual energy and a decreased need for sleep. Hypomania often precedes the onset of mania.
- **Mania** In mania all, or many, of the symptoms associated with hypomania will be evident but there may also be psychotic symptoms such as grandiose delusions and/ or also auditory hallucinations. Damaging, inappropriate actions, such as spending excessive sums of money, or aggression often occur as a result of psychotic symptoms. Speech is often rapid and difficult to follow and concentration intermittent.

ASSESSMENT

Assess for elevation of mood, overtalkativeness, flight of ideas, increased physical and mental efficiency, disruption of social and work relationships, increased energy, overfamiliarity. In mania, assess for pressure of speech, inability to sustain attention, inflated self-esteem, grandiose ideas. Mood may be suspicious and irritable. Mania may occur with or without psychotic symptoms. Assess for the presence of psychotic symptoms such as grandiose or religious delusions; marked flight of ideas and pressure of speech may result in the person becoming incomprehensible. Severe and sustained physical activity or excitement may result in aggressive behaviour, and neglect of eating, drinking and personal hygiene. Delusions and hallucinations can be mood congruent or incongruent.

POSSIBLE PROBES

Probes should be used in history taking, such as:

- Have you felt more confident or happier recently?
- Have you had more ideas or thoughts than usual?
- Are you more irritable than normal?
- Have you been more flirtatious than usual, or been overspending?

FACTFILE

1. An estimated 60% of patients with affective disorders also have comorbid substance misuse.
2. Physical health needs must also be met; risks of overactivity and poor nutrition; also check for hyperthyroidism.
3. Mania with psychotic symptoms may be difficult to differentiate from schizophrenia.
4. Treatment: inpatient care, sometimes under the Mental Health Act, sedation (e.g. benzodiazepine), antipsychotic and mood stabilizers usually required.

DEPRESSIVE EPISODE/DISORDER ★★★★★

Depressive disorder is a common diagnosis and there is a good chance of it occurring in a clinical examination. In OSCEs it is unlikely that a student would be expected to diagnose a comorbid depressive condition, with schizophrenia or alcoholism, within the time available; however, more complex comorbid scenarios could well occur in long case examinations.

DEFINITIONS

- **Dysthymia** A chronic depression of mood that does not currently fulfil criteria for recurrent depressive disorder.
- **Mild, moderate or severe depressive episodes** Depressed mood, loss of interest and enjoyment, increased fatigue, combined with reduced concentration, self-esteem, self-confidence, disturbed sleep, reduced appetite and weight loss, negative ideas about self and the future.
- **Postnatal depression** Depressive episode occurring soon after childbirth.

ASSESSMENT

In some cases individuals with depression will offer explanations as to why they believe they have become depressed, but are also likely to manifest biological or cognitive symptoms. Some patients will not complain of depressed mood, saying instead they are failing to cope, feel a failure in some way or feel excessively fatigued. Many depressed individuals will not report significant life events before the onset of their condition.

POSSIBLE PROBES

- How do you feel in your mood or spirits?
- Have you felt that things were getting on top of you?
- Do you feel a failure or guilty?
- Ask about sleep, appetite, weight and concentration.
- Ask about past medical and family history.

INVESTIGATIONS

These should be undertaken to exclude organic causes (e.g. FBC, biochemistry, ESR, blood glucose, thyroid function, chest X-ray).

FACTFILE

1. According to the World Health Organization, depression is the number one cause of global morbidity. They estimate that around 340 million people worldwide have depressive disorder.
2. Depressive disorder is more prevalent among women than men: an estimated 7–12% of men suffer during their life and roughly 20–25% of women.
3. Approximately 10–20% of children need help for depressive disorder.
4. 15% of those diagnosed with depressive disorder in the UK commit suicide.
5. Family doctors are said to recognize about 50% of depressive disorder.
6. Depression may present as cognitive impairment in over-65s (so-called 'pseudodementia').

DELIBERATE SELF-HARM AND SUICIDE ★★★★★

You may well be asked to assess the risk of suicide or further self-harm in a patient who has recently attempted suicide or self-harmed, because such patients present frequently. It is therefore imperative that you are able to assess and discuss the management of such individuals, as they form common OSCE scenarios.

DEFINITIONS

- **Attempted suicide**   An attempt to take one's own life.
- **Deliberate self-harm**   Non-fatal acts of self-injury.
- **Parasuicide**   An apparent attempt to commit suicide.
- **Suicide**   A willful, self-inflicted, life-threatening act that results in death.

ASSESSMENT

- Take note of significant recent stress or loss.
- Note actions that suggest intent to commit suicide, such as hoarding tablets and alcohol, leaving a note of suicidal intent, putting affairs in order and arranging to be alone for a significant period of time during the attempt.
- Assess for coexisting mental illness, precipitating or provoking events, distress at the time, substance abuse at the time, previous history of self-harm.
- History of past psychiatric disorders (e.g. affective illness, schizophrenia, alcoholism, personality disorder)?
- History of self-harm?
- Suicidal thoughts?
- Inability to think about the future?
- Any of the symptoms of depression as listed above?
- Physical evidence of self-harm, e.g. scars on forearms?

POSSIBLE PROBES

- Have you ever felt that your problems have become too much to cope with?
- Do you still feel like this?

- Have you ever thought that it would be a relief not to wake up?
- Have you ever considered taking your own life? (Do you still feel like this?)
- Have you ever planned to take your own life? (Do you still have such plans?)

FACTFILE

1. 70% of suicides in the UK are by people who are depressed.
2. Other mental health disorders, such as depression, psychosis or substance misuse, increase the chance of suicide.
3. Single men are most likely to attempt suicide, and other socio-economic factors, such as unemployment or isolation in a deprived urban area, are identified risk factors.
4. Deliberate self-harm accounts for an estimated 10% of acute medical admissions.
5. Parasuicide is 30 times more common than suicide.

ANXIETY-BASED DISORDERS ★★★★★

Traditionally referred to as neuroses, these disorders are evidenced by excessive concern or anxiety that has a debilitating affect upon the individual's daily life. There is usually an accompanying set of somatic symptoms due to autonomic arousal. Keep in mind that many people with depressive disorder also show excessive anxiety.

POST-TRAUMATIC STRESS DISORDER ★★★

DEFINITION

A condition precipitated by experience of a life-threatening, or other extremely stressful, event. There is a definite history of some sort of major trauma that appears to be a clear provoking factor. There may be a delay of several months before the patient presents, but the trauma is usually recent.

KEY CLINICAL FEATURES

- Classic signs of anxiety (see below).
- Nightmares.
- Flashbacks (intrusive memories) with associated fear/panic.
- Hypervigilance, increased startle response.
- Avoidance of stimuli/situations associated with the trauma.
- Other coping strategies, such as reliance on alcohol or drugs.

ASSESSMENT

- Ask about effects of the stressful situation.
- Symptoms are often associated with autonomic arousal and insomnia.
- Anxiety and depression may also occur.
- Onset follows the trauma, often with a latency period of weeks to months.
- Recovery is expected in most cases; some cases becoming chronic.

POSSIBLE PROBES

- How were you before (the trauma)?
- How have you been since (the trauma)?

FACTFILE

1. Approximately 5% of men and 11% of women are affected by PTSD at some point during their life.

2. Less severe cases can recover fully within 3 months.
3. More severe cases and/or treatment delay can result in chronic PTSD.
4. Treatment often involves a combination of antidepressant drug(s) and CBT.

PANIC DISORDERS ★★★

DEFINITION

Unpredictable, recurrent episodes of severe anxiety that are not associated with a particular situation or set of circumstances.

KEY CLINICAL FEATURES

Panic disorders regularly present with phobic disorders, or a history of them, or with depression. Symptoms must have persisted for a minimum of 1 month, cause substantial distress and impair function. Attacks usually last only minutes.

ASSESSMENT

- Somatic symptoms (sudden onset)
- Feelings of unreality (depersonalization or derealization)
- Subjective discomfort
- Fear of losing control, or dying, or going mad
- Feelings of impending danger or apprehension
- Constant and exhausting alertness
- Fear of further panic attacks
- Sweating
- Palpitations, chest pain
- Hyperventilation or shortness of breath

- Nausea, choking sensation
- Hot flushes
- Lightheadedness or feeling faint
- Trembling

POSSIBLE PROBES

- Do you ever feel you may lose control during an attack? What are you afraid would happen?
- Does a fear of becoming anxious make you avoid certain situations?

A history of unpredictable anxiety attacks and the above symptoms give clues to diagnosis.

INVESTIGATIONS

These are those required to exclude organic causes such as hyperthyroidism, phaeochromocytoma (rarely), ischaemic heart disease and hypoglycaemia.

FACTFILE

1. 15% of those with general anxiety, or panic, disorders have a first-degree relative with a similar difficulty.
2. Females account for two-thirds of those with panic disorders.
3. Patients often think that their panic attacks last for an extended period of time. In fact, they rarely last longer than a few minutes.
4. Antidepressants are often effective for panic disorders.
5. Beta blockers such as propranolol can help reduce somatic symptoms.

PHOBIC ANXIETY DISORDERS ★★★

DEFINITIONS

In this group of disorders, anxiety occurs in certain well-defined situations, which are not currently thought to be dangerous. Phobic anxiety is indistinguishable, behaviourally and physiologically, from other types of anxiety. It often coexists with depression.

- **Agoraphobia** Fear not only of open spaces but of crowds, and the inability to escape quickly to a safer place. May overlap with fears of leaving home, or entering crowded places. Often presents with panic disorder, or with a history of panic disorder.
- **Social phobia** Fear of scrutiny by others in small groups, usually leading to social isolation. May be restricted to, for example, eating out in public, meeting the opposite sex, etc. Social phobias are associated with fear of embarrassment, introversion, self-doubt and persistent concerns about the view of others. They often present as a fear of blushing and/or tremor in company. Avoidance is often marked, leading to social isolation.

ASSESSMENT

The psychological, behavioural or autonomic symptoms must be primarily related to anxiety and not secondary to other problems such as delusions. The anxiety should be restricted to the phobic situation. There will also be marked avoidance of the phobic situation. A family history of anxiety disorders, overprotection during childhood, parental attitudes and anxiety during childhood appear to be important.

POSSIBLE PROBES

- Do you find that particular situations, surroundings or objects make you more nervous than normal?
- What do you think is the worst thing that could happen in such a situation?
- Do you actively avoid certain situations? (If so, which ones?)

FACTFILE

1. Onset is normally in childhood or early adult life.
2. Some medicines, such as diazepam, can be successfully used in the short-term to alleviate anxiety, but regular use may lead to dependence.
3. Antidepressants are commonly used to treat phobic anxiety disorders.
4. Psychological interventions, including so-called 'graded exposure' and CBT are commonly used.

OBSESSIVE–COMPULSIVE DISORDER ★★★★

DEFINITION

Recurrent obsessional thoughts or compulsive actions that cause distress and interfere with normal life. The ideas are recognized as the person's own and normally seen to be irrational, and resisted unsuccessfully.

ASSESSMENT

- Repetitive, unpleasant or intrusive thoughts, images or impulses that enter the individual's mind in a stereotyped form and are experienced against conscious resistance. Almost always distressing, e.g. violent or obscene.

- Compulsive acts or rituals are stereotyped behaviours that are repeated again and again. They are not enjoyable, but usually aimed at preventing some unlikely event. Common examples include examples of compulsive behaviour: washing hands over and over again (fear of contamination); other complex rituals to do with cleanliness; arranging objects in order that they conform to a particular pattern; repeating words or actions a particular number of times (to prevent some ill consequence); checking switches, lights or locks numerous times (not just two or three); compulsion to think about ideas or images (e.g. obscenities).
- Autonomic anxiety symptoms often may be present.
- There is a close relationship between OCD and depressive disorder (often depressive symptoms are present).
- Impaired functioning due to compulsions may severely affect life style (e.g. cleaning rituals can take hours).

POSSIBLE PROBES

- Do you find yourself checking things repeatedly? (How often?)
- Do you like things especially clean and tidy or in a particular order?
- Do you ever try to resist having these thoughts or doing these things?

FACTFILE

1. Onset is usually in childhood or early adult life.
2. Obsessional personality types are at increased risk of OCD.
3. OCD is probably more common in men than women.
4. Prevalence is around 1 in 1000 people.

ORGANIC DISORDERS ★★★★
ACUTE CONFUSION/DELIRIUM ★★★
DEFINITION

An aetiologically non-specific syndrome characterized by disturbances of consciousness and attention, perception, thinking, memory, psychomotor behaviour, emotion and the sleep–wake cycle.

KEY CLINICAL FEATURES

- May occur at any age, but commoner over 60 years.
- Onset usually rapid.
- Transient and fluctuating intensity.
- Variable duration (days/weeks/months).

ASSESSMENT

- Full physical examination and investigation is necessary to establish the underlying cause.
- Impairment of consciousness (from clouding to coma).
- Inability to focus, sustain, shift attention.
- Global disturbance of cognitive function (disorientation – time, place, person).
- Perceptual distortion (illusions and often visual hallucinations).
- Psychomotor disturbance (hypo- or hyperactivity).
- Sleep–wake cycle disturbed (e.g. insomnia).
- Emotional disturbance (e.g. anxiety, fear, euphoria).

FACTFILE

1. Common causes: UTI, chronic liver disease, carcinoma, sub-acute bacterial endocarditis.
2. Management best sited within a medical unit with psychiatric input.

DEMENTIAS ★★★★

A group of diseases that impair brain functions from a previous level of functioning. All dementias involve memory loss, but other cognitive deficits occur, including agnosia, aphasia and loss of executive function. Dementia results from irreversible changes to the brain caused by cerebrovascular disease (multi-infarct dementia, MID), infection (e.g. HIV, CJD, syphilis), trauma or degenerative processes such as AD.

KEY CLINICAL FEATURES

- Onset is often gradual, first indication may be memory difficulties or a change in personality.
- Impaired judgement, loss of social graces.
- Impaired personal hygiene or appearance.
- If delirium is present, dementia cannot be diagnosed, although, in patients with established dementia, delirium can coexist, for example due to UTI.
- In later stages, paranoid ideas and delusions can occur.
- Restlessness, wandering.
- Memory impairment. In mild dementia this may only involve recent memory, producing disorientation; however, as dementia worsens, remote memory is also affected.
- Behaviour and/or personality changes.

POSSIBLE PROBES

- Have you experienced any difficulties with your memory recently?
- Can I ask you one or two questions we ask everyone? (Good introduction to using the MMSE.)
- Can you tell me the year and the month? What is the name of the Prime Minister?

ALZHEIMER'S DISEASE ★★★★

DEFINITION

Alzheimer's disease is the commonest form of dementia and it occurs predominantly amongst those aged 65 and over; incidence increases steadily with age. A definitive diagnosis requires postmortem neuropathological investigation, showing plaques and neurofibrillary tangles in affected brain areas.

KEY CLINICAL FEATURES

- AD is gradual and progressive.
- In over 50% of patients (recent) memory loss is the first symptom.
- Dyspraxias present as dressing difficulties or trouble with route finding.
- Dysphasia may appear as word finding difficulties.
- Agnosias may initially appear as trouble recognizing a new acquaintance.
- Some patients with AD will show perceptual defects, such as illusions or hallucinations; many may also become suspicious or paranoid, especially in later stages.
- At least 20% of AD sufferers become depressed.

ASSESSMENT

Diagnosis of AD is inferred from the absence of other causes for the dementia. It is essential to eliminate other treatable causes, including cerebrovascular disease, hypothyroidism, vitamin B_{12} deficiency, anaemia and depression. Assessment requires a full physical assessment, cognitive testing (e.g. MMSE) and brain imaging.

1. AD is more common among women than men.
2. Around 5% of AD occurs in individuals under 65 years.
3. Approximately 500 000 people in Britain have AD. Worldwide there are around 12 million sufferers.
4. Multidisciplinary assessment and case management is essential.

LEWY BODY DEMENTIA ★★

DEFINITION

Dementia caused by presence of Lewy bodies in the brain, producing characteristic clinical features.

KEY CLINICAL FEATURES

- Development of dementia with many features overlapping those of AD, especially impaired recent memory.
- Development of parkinsonism.
- Fluctuation in severity of the condition from day to day.
- Early development of complex visual hallucinations.
- Cognitive impairment can be mild in some cases.
- Tendency to falls.

ASSESSMENT

- Exclude treatable causes.
- There are no specific diagnostic tests for LBD; diagnosis is inferred from clinical features and confirmed by post-mortem examination.

- Detailed psychometric and clinical assessments are necessary.
- Neuroimaging may be helpful.

MULTI-INFARCT DEMENTIA ★★★★

DEFINITION

MID or vascular dementia typically develops through a series of small decrements in function as mini-strokes occur in the brain.

KEY CLINICAL FEATURES

- Memory loss.
- Impaired executive function.
- Apathy.
- Emotional liability.
- Deterioration in personal care.
- There may be a history of cardio/cerebrovascular disease.

ASSESSMENT

- Assess CVS and CNS (hypertension, focal neurological signs of stroke, etc.).
- CXR and ECG may be useful. Neuroimaging maybe helpful.

FACTFILE

1. Approximately 20% of dementias have a vascular origin.
2. Likelihood increases if the patient has hypertension or diabetes.
3. Management: control contributing physical illness; low-dose aspirin may be useful.

EATING DISORDERS ★★★

ANOREXIA NERVOSA ★★★

DEFINITION

Significant and deliberate loss of body weight (at least 15%, usually through a deliberate restriction in intake of calories) accompanied by a distorted body image, where patients view themselves as fat, even though they are often very thin.

KEY CLINICAL FEATURES

- May well have a comorbid depressive or obsessive disorder.
- Patient will not maintain minimum body weight.
- A fear of weight gain, despite being underweight.
- Distorted self-perception of body shape or weight.
- Denial of seriousness of low weight.
- Female patients will have missed three or more periods due to weight loss.
- Attempts to conceal the eating disorder.
- Desire to exert control over his or her life.
- Social withdrawal.
- Undernourished, tired and may feel cold.
- Low blood pressure.

ASSESSMENT

A collateral history is essential, as individuals often present because friends or family have concerns. Full mental and physical examination and weight monitoring (BMI). May need admission to specialized inpatient unit.

POSSIBLE PROBES

- Do you feel that your eating habits require control?
- Do you worry about weight gain or getting fat?

- Have you ever used medicines (e.g. laxatives), or made yourself sick, to control your weight?
- (Females) When was your last period?
- Have you ever eaten in binges?
- How much exercise do you take?

FACTFILE

1. Affects less than 1% of the female population.
2. 5% of patients die of complications.

BULIMIA NERVOSA ★★★

DEFINITION

Bulimia nervosa refers to repetitive and excessive binge eating. To prevent body weight and shape ballooning, compensatory vomiting or use of laxatives or diuretics occurs. It is associated with a disproportionate emphasis upon body shape and body weight, although there is no distorted self-image, as occurs in anorexia nervosa. The age of presentation is often later than in anorexia.

KEY CLINICAL FEATURES

- BMI often within normal limits.
- May have a comorbid anxiety or depressive disorder.
- Perception of self is disproportionately related to body shape and weight.
- Binge eating and inappropriate weight control measures (e.g. laxatives, exercise, self-induced vomiting) more than twice a week.
- Hoarse voice.
- Renal failure.
- Teeth affected by gastric acid.

ASSESSMENT

- Full physical and mental state examination.
- Correct physical complications such as electrolyte imbalance.
- Take a careful history of binge eating and weight control measures.
- Identify any morbid dread of fatness.

POSSIBLE PROBES

- Do you ever feel that your eating habits are out of control?
- Have you ever binged on food?
- Have you ever controlled your weight by vomiting, laxatives or excessive exercise?

FACTFILE

1. It is estimated that around 2% of all women aged between 16 and 35 have, or have had, bulimia nervosa.
2. There is often an earlier history of anorexia nervosa.

PERSONALITY AND/OR BEHAVIOURAL DISORDERS ★★★

Personality disorders are a group of conditions that describe ingrained, dysfunctional and inflexible responses. They represent significant deviations from the way the average individual in a given culture thinks, feels and relates to others. The individual with a personality disorder shows long-term functioning that is maladaptive, to the extent that it causes subjective distress and/or impairs occupational or social functioning.

DISSOCIAL (PSYCHOPATHIC) PERSONALITY DISORDER ★★★

KEY CLINICAL FEATURES

- Irresponsible and antisocial behaviour.
- Functioning tends to improve with age.
- Occupational disruption.
- Promiscuity.
- Violent and aggressive.
- Impulsive behaviour; needing immediate gratification.

ANXIOUS (AVOIDANT) PERSONALITY DISORDER ★★

KEY CLINICAL FEATURES

- Persistent feelings of tension and apprehension.
- Avoidance of social/personal contact.
- Fear of rejection and criticism.

BORDERLINE (EMOTIONALLY UNSTABLE) PERSONALITY DISORDER ★★★

KEY CLINICAL FEATURES

- History of turbulent relationships with others.
- Impulsivity.
- Mood swings.
- Psychotic-like symptoms, often stress-induced.
- Repeated behavioural crises.

DEPENDENT PERSONALITY DISORDER ★★

KEY CLINICAL FEATURES

- Excessively dependent upon others for praise and reassurance.
- Exaggerated, emotional symptoms, associated with histrionic personality disorder, are not evident.

HISTRIONIC PERSONALITY DISORDER ★

KEY CLINICAL FEATURES

- Excessive emotionality.
- Pervasive attention-seeking behaviour, such as demanding praise, reassurance or approval.
- Flamboyant behaviour.
- Shallow, transient emotions.

NARCISSISTIC PERSONALITY DISORDER ★

KEY CLINICAL FEATURES

- Excessively self-centred.
- Egotistical.
- Prone to intense jealousy.

PARANOID PERSONALITY DISORDER ★★★

KEY CLINICAL FEATURES

- Persistent and unprovoked inclination to perceive others' actions as being threatening, without any sufficient basis for these beliefs (paranoid ideation).
- General expectation of being exploited in some way (distrust).
- Psychotic symptoms, such as hallucinations or delusions, are never part of paranoid personality disorder, although they may be evident in a comorbid condition.
- Oversensitive to criticism.
- Self-importance and stubbornness.

SCHIZOID PERSONALITY DISORDER ★★

KEY CLINICAL FEATURES

- Restricted emotional range and expression.
- Emotional detachment.

- Indifference to social relationships, sexual or otherwise, often including family.
- Indifferent attitude towards others.

Symptoms are often evident by adolescence or early adulthood and continue throughout adult life. Nonetheless, they usually become less pronounced in middle or old age. Individuals with a personality disorder may well present with complaints of depression or anxiety, the root cause of which are egosyntonic or egodystonic traits.

Remember that abnormal personality traits (e.g. anxiety) are distinct from the diagnosis of a personality disorder. Asking the patient to make substantive comparisons with a period when they were well can help to identify changes quickly, and therefore help decide which type of personality disorder the patient may have.

ASSESSMENT

Personality disorders rarely require hospitalization. The main exceptions to this are when there is a comorbid disorder, such as major depression or substance misuse. In severe cases of dissocial or borderline personality disorder short-term admission may be necessary to assess further or defuse a situation.

Often an individual will not fall neatly into one specific personality disorder category and may present with symptoms associated with a combination of traits.

POSSIBLE PROBES

- Is the patient a shy person or a 'worrier' (anxious)?
- How does the individual respond to criticism (anxious or paranoid)?
- How does the patient get on with people (paranoid)?
- Does he or she trust other people (paranoid or schizoid)?

- Could the patient be described as a loner (schizoid)?
- To what extent does this patient depend upon others (dependent)?
- Is the patient impulsive (emotionally unstable)?
- What is his or her temper like (dissocial)?
- Is the patient dramatic or irresponsible (dissocial or histrionic)?
- Does the patient have unusually high standards at work or at home (obsessional)?

FACTFILE

1. Some personality disorders have distinct but related diagnoses for children and adolescents (usually under 18s). For example, conduct disorder in children has similarities to dissocial personality disorder; in fact for a diagnosis of dissocial personality disorder to be made the individual should have a history of conduct disorder before the age of 15.

2. Dissocial personality disorder is five times more likely to occur in those who have a similarly affected male first-degree blood relative. If the first-degree relative with the condition is female, the likelihood increases to ten times more likely.

Discussion point

There is no specific treatment for personality disorders. Treatment tends to be targeted at problem or symptom areas. Some forms of psychological treatment, such as CBT or psychotherapy, or medication may be helpful in some cases. It is essential that clear expectations are given about what health professionals can and cannot offer the patient. It is also essential that staff emphasize what is expected of the patient. People with a personality disorder often present out of hours in crisis and can cause considerable concern because of the risks to themselves or others.

SCHIZOPHRENIA AND RELATED PSYCHOSES ★★★★★

See also mania and depressive psychosis, discussed earlier in this chapter.

SCHIZOPHRENIA ★★★★★

Schizophrenia is the most common psychotic disorder and is seen in all cultures. It occurs with an incidence of about 2–4 per 10000 per year, with a lifetime risk of about 1%. In 1990 the World Health Organization examined the occurrence of schizophrenia in 10 different countries and found that the incidence of broadly defined schizophrenia varied by a factor of four. There appears to be equal lifetime risk for both sexes, although the peak age of onset is 15–25 for men and 25–35 for women.

DEFINITION

Schizophrenia is a group of disorders with the following features: abnormal thoughts (e.g. delusions), disorders of thought process and speech (e.g. loosening of associations), abnormal perceptions (e.g. hallucinations), abnormal affect (flat or incongruous), passivity phenomena (e.g. thought insertion or broadcasting), cognitive impairments, and lack of insight. Schizophrenia is a neurodevelopmental disorder that is the result of a combination of genetic and environmental factors.

KEY CLINICAL FEATURES

A number of different groups of symptoms occur, including positive, negative, affective and impairments of cognition. Positive symptoms are additional to the normal mental state (e.g. hallucinations), while negative symptoms represent a reduction in normal features (e.g. psychomotor poverty).

Positive symptoms
- Formal thought disorder.
- Disorganized behaviour.
- Inappropriate affect.
- Delusions.
- Hallucinations (e.g. hearing voices).

Negative symptoms
- Poverty of thought and speech.
- Impaired volition.
- Blunted affect.
- Social withdrawal.

Cognitive impairments
- Poor concentration and memory.
- Poor speech (content) and/or decision-making ability.

HISTORY

Often schizophrenia is precipitated by a traumatic event or stressful period.

There is strong evidence that genetic factors play a role in schizophrenia. The psychiatric history of relatives, particularly first-degree relatives, is therefore important. While some individuals do recover from schizophrenia, for most it is a lifelong affliction.

Certain delusions are more commonly observed in schizophrenia than in other psychotic disorders. These include thought broadcasting, thought insertion, thought withdrawal and delusions of being controlled.

ASSESSMENT

Be wary about diagnosing schizophrenia if the cause of the psychosis is:

- schizoaffective or a mood disorder
- personality disorder
- a medical condition
- substance misuse.

POSSIBLE PROBES

- Do you think that people are planning to harm you?
- Are people plotting against you?
- Do you ever hear or see things that others do not?
- Have you ever heard voices when there was nobody about?

Do remember that schizophrenia may occur with the above conditions. None of the symptoms present in schizophrenia are found solely in patients with schizophrenia, e.g. hallucinations occur in many different conditions. Schizophrenia may present with predominantly positive or predominantly negative symptoms, or a mixture of both.

FACTFILE

1. 22% of those who experience a single acute episode will fully recover.
2. 35% who experience several acute episodes will have no, or minimal, social impairment.
3. 35% will have worsening social impairment following each acute episode, with no return to normality.

DISCUSSION POINTS

1. *Medication.* What are most appropriate medications for positive symptoms? Do antipsychotics help negative symptoms? When might you prescribe a benzodiazepine or clozapine? Describe the main side effects of specific antipsychotic drugs.

2. *Psychological and social aspects of treatment.* Recognize the importance of CBT and social interventions for the management of schizophrenia. Many people with schizophrenia require long-term multidisciplinary support.

SCHIZOAFFECTIVE DISORDER ★★★★★

DEFINITION

Some people show significant features of both schizophrenia and affective disorder during a single episode of illness and are therefore classified as having 'schizoaffective disorder'.

KEY CLINICAL FEATURES

- Mood and schizophrenic symptoms are both present (see above).
- The prognosis of schizoaffective disorder appears to lie between schizophrenia and affective disorder.

Discussion point

Treatment targets mood and psychotic symptoms; antipsychotics are often combined with mood stabilizers.

DELUSIONAL DISORDERS ★★★

DEFINITION

This term refers to patients who show delusional symptoms in the absence of significant other mood or schizophrenic symptoms.

KEY CLINICAL FEATURES

- Symptoms should have persisted for a minimum of 1 month.

- Onset is usually in middle age, although it can be earlier.
- Affective, organic and schizophrenic symptoms are absent.
- Delusions are often not bizarre and are often persecutory (or paranoid), but can also be of morbid jealousy, erotomania or somatic, e.g. monosymptomatic hypochondriacal delusions.
- The content of the delusions varies hugely but often relates to the patient's life, e.g. litigation, or that others think they are homosexual.
- Function and behaviour remain unimpaired.
- No major mood disturbance or negative symptoms.
- Delusions may be systematized or encapsulated (circumscribed).

DISCUSSION POINT

Do not diagnose delusional disorder if other symptoms associated with schizophrenia are present. Treatment is usually with antipsychotic drugs with variable success, depending on the duration of symptoms before treatment started. The management of the risk associated with the delusions is important, e.g. in a patient with delusions of morbid jealousy about a partner.

SUBSTANCE MISUSE AND ADDICTION ★★★★
DEFINITIONS

Substance misuse occurs when substances taken for pleasure cause physical, psychological or social harm. *Addiction* is defined as dependence, both physiological and psychological, on a particular substance, such as alcohol or another drug. *Dependence* on a substance leads to withdrawal symptoms when that substance is discontinued. Dependence on alcohol is termed alcoholism. After taking a drug, *acute intoxication* can occur leading to drunkenness in the case of alcohol, or psychosis in the case of amphetamines or hallucinogens like LSD.

Commonly more than one drug is abused (polydrug abuse). Sometimes patients with other mental health problems also misuse drugs e.g. bipolar patients sometimes abuse alcohol while people with schizophrenia may abuse cannabis; this is referred to as *dual diagnosis*. Alcohol and/or drug misuse or addiction can also be associated with a personality disorder, anxiety disorder or affective illness.

HISTORY

This is directed at identifying the degree of dependence and the adverse outcomes (psychological, physical, social) associated with this.

ASSESSMENT

- Know the features of misuse of alcohol and other commonly used drugs.
- Know the physical and psychiatric conditions associated with substance misuse.
- Physical examination essential.
- A good history will help identify and quantify the substance being misused (e.g. Units of alcohol per week).
- Alcohol can be measured in breath or blood and many other substances can be measured in a urine sample e.g. benzodiazepines, opioids, amphetamines, LSD and cannabis.
- Ask every patient about alcohol and other substance misuse.

COMMONLY MISUSED SUBSTANCES
ALCOHOL ★★★★★

Harmful use may cause physical, psychiatric and social problems. The student should be familiar with the harmful effects of alcohol misuse including physical, neurological, psychiatric, family and social complications. Dependence (alcoholism) requires: a compulsion to drink, increased tolerance to effects of alcohol, drinking to relieve withdrawal symptoms, withdrawal symptoms, primacy of drinking in person's lifestyle.

Withdrawal provokes tremulousness, agitation, cravings, and sweating. The most severe withdrawal syndrome is delirium tremens (the 'DTs'): occurs 24–48 hours after stopping heavy drinking, clouded consciousness (delirium), visual hallucinations or illusions, paranoid ideation, fearfulness, tremor, autonomic arousal (sweating, pyrexia, tachycardia, hypertension), insomnia, dehydration. Be able to distinguish DTs from *alcoholic hallucinosis*. Ten percent of people with alcoholism commit suicide.

CANNABIS ★★★★

Widely used drug from *Cannabis sativa* plant with many active constituents including THC (tetrahydrocannabinol). Effects include: impairment of motor and cognitive performance, increased feelings of calmness and contentedness, space/time distortions. Some users experience anxiety or paranoid ideation. No withdrawal syndrome but tolerance can occur. Cannabis is considered a risk factor for schizophrenia.

OPIOIDS ★★★★

A highly addictive group that includes heroin, morphine, methadone and codeine. The opioids can be injected intravenously (associated with infection risk (HIV, Hep B and C), phlebitis and thrombosis), inhaled or snorted. Opioids produce a feeling of euphoria, but regular use produces marked tolerance. Cessation provokes a severe withdrawal syndrome usually within 8–10 hours of the last dose.

STIMULANTS ★★★

The main members of this group include the amphetamines, 3,4-methylenedioxymetamphetamine (MDMA, ecstasy), cocaine, and phencyclidine (PCP). Most stimulants produce feelings of well-being, increased motor activity, insomnia and elation through stimulation of brain mono-aminergic systems, although PCP antagonizes NMDA receptors. The stimulants are addictive and rapidly induce tolerance. In some people a paranoid psychosis develops. Withdrawal may provoke depression and suicidal thoughts. Ecstasy appears to cause massive 5HT release resulting in elation, hallucinosis and excessive, repetitive motor behaviour that may explain its wide use in UK dance clubs.

HALLUCINOGENS ★★★

Members of this group include the synthetic lysergic acid diethylamide (LSD) and psilocybin (from 'magic mushrooms'). Effects include perceptual change (often illusions), heightened sensory perception e.g. of sounds, visual distortions, hallucinosis and intense euphoria. Sometimes after stopping the hallucinogen, the patient re-experiences the altered perception that occurred while intoxicated (flashback). Some patients find flashbacks very distressing.

Other drugs of misuse include solvents (especially in younger people), benzodiazepines (prescribed or non-prescribed), anabolic steroids (athletes and body-builders), nicotine and caffeine.

INDEX